PALEO ICE CREAM

PALEO ICE CREAM

75 RECIPES FOR RICH AND CREAMY HOMEMADE SCOOPS AND TREATS

BEN HIRSHBERG

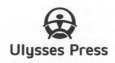

Ulysses Press

Published by
Ulysses Press
P.O. Box 3440
Berkeley, CA 94703
www.ulyssespress.com

ISBN: 978-1-61243-352-3
Library of Congress Catalog Number 2014932308

Printed in the United States by Bang Printing

10 9 8 7 6 5 4 3 2 1

Acquisitions editor: Kelly Reed
Managing editor: Claire Chun
Project editor: Alice Riegert
Editor: Beverly McGuire
Proofreader: Renee Rutledge
Front cover design/interior layout and design: what!design @ whatweb.com
Cover photography: vanilla ice cream © dana2000/shutterstock.com, chocolate
   ice cream © tacar/shutterstock.com, green tea Ice cream © Piyato/shutterstock.
   com, strawberry ice cream © Christian Jung/shutterstock.com; strawberry
   cheesecake ice cream © MaraZe/shutterstock.com; coffee ice cream © Kati
   Molin/shutterstock.com; blueberry sorbet © verca/shutterstock.com

Distributed by Publishers Group West

*For my dad, Rich; my mom, Wendi; my girlfriend, Kelsey;
and all of the other good people out there.*

TABLE OF CONTENTS

INTRODUCTION

Paleo ice cream. On its face, it sounds like an oxymoron. What kind of purportedly healthy diet includes ice cream!? It sounds even more heinous when you examine the concept of paleo. Our ancestors from the Paleolithic era certainly weren't chowing down on fudge bars. So what gives?

The paleo concept is interpreted differently by different people. Some paleo folks believe that followers of the diet should completely abstain from eating anything that was not eaten 10,000 years ago. Others believe that paleo eaters should consume only meat and vegetables while restricting carbohydrate intake. Still other paleo supporters think that the paleo diet is just a template from which to work and that the focus should be on eating whole foods rather than on restriction. I fall into the last camp. I believe that the purpose of paleo is not to try and reenact life from the Paleolithic era. For me, eating paleo is instead about consuming the whole, nutrient-dense foods that we evolved to eat.

Viewed in that light, ice cream can very much be included in one's diet so long as it is made up of nutritious ingredients. That is where things get tricky, though, because most store-bought ice cream is made from very processed, nutrient-poor ingredients.

I know this all too well, because I still ate store-bought ice cream before writing this cookbook. Being a health nerd, I would always read the ingredient list on the back of the carton. It isn't pretty. Milk that probably came from sick, sedentary cows; lots of refined, white sugar; and a long list of chemicals that I couldn't pronounce. Yikes! But what was I to do? I love my ice cream!

One beautiful spring day, my girlfriend, Kelsey, surprised me with a picnic lunch in the Washington Park Arboretum. For our main course, we had the usual fare: spaghetti squash with ground beef marinara sauce and a kale-strawberry salad. But the dessert blew my mind. It was homemade Chai Tea Ice Cream (the very same recipe included in this book on page 54).

First of all, how does one bring ice cream to a picnic and keep it frozen? Second, it tasted amazing! Then she told me it was PALEO ice cream. As we ate the whole container and licked the lid, Kelsey told me all about how she used coconut milk, honey, and egg yolks for the ice cream base. For the rest of the day, my mind was spinning thinking about all of the recipes I could try using Kelsey's ice cream base recipe.

And try them I did. That summer I made ice cream several times a week, and sometimes multiple times a day. I couldn't resist the ice cream experimentation. At the end of the summer I self-published an eBook containing all of my favorite recipes, and many people loved it. Some were left wanting more recipes, though, so I went back to work.

Partway through my revamping process, Ulysses Press emailed me and told me they'd like to acquire my title. The timing was perfect! The lovely folks at Ulysses helped me focus where I needed to focus and add where I needed to add; they even gave me flavor suggestions.

What you are holding is the culmination of my ice cream escapades: a collection of ice cream recipes that are not only extremely tasty, but also full of whole food ingredients and plentiful in the essential nutrients needed for us to live healthfully.

So no, cavemen probably didn't eat ice cream, contrary to what you would believe if you watched Fred Flintstone run around in his ice cream truck. But if you view paleo as a diet made up of nutritious whole foods, then ice cream can fit into that box quite nicely. That's right: ice cream can be a healthy dessert option if it is made with nourishing ingredients. So throw off the bowlines, sail away from the harbor, catch the trade winds in your sails. And make some ice cream!

HOW TO USE THIS BOOK

This book contains three main types of ice cream recipes: traditional, banana, and cashew. The banana and cashew butter recipes are quite straightforward: they are made with a base of either bananas or cashew butter. There isn't too much wiggle room for ingredient substitution and tweaking. Sure, you can increase or decrease quantities of ingredients or maybe substitute certain supporting ingredients. But the base of those recipes will always be bananas or cashew butter.

This is not so for the more traditional recipes. For these recipes, the ice cream base can be tweaked quite extensively, and it is in your best interest to customize the recipes to make them exactly how you want them. What follows is a quick primer on how to best make the traditional ice cream recipes for your preferences and needs.

SUBSTITUTIONS

ICE CREAM BASES

To start, you should know that you can substitute any dairy product or dairy alternative for the one listed in the recipe. For example, in the Vanilla Ice Cream recipe (page 19), I list coconut milk as the main base ingredient. If you don't like how coconut milk tastes, you can substitute any nut milk, or if you eat dairy, cream, or half and half. It all depends on how well your body and taste buds tolerate certain ingredients. Here is a quick rundown of all of the dairy products and dairy alternatives:

FULL-FAT COCONUT MILK: This is usually sold in cans and is probably the most commonly used paleo ice cream base. It has plenty of healthy fats, so it is rich and thick, just like the cream and milk used in traditional ice cream. Its flavor is too much for some people, adored by others, and can be masked by strong flavors such as mint extract, coffee, and so on.

ALMOND MILK AND REDUCED-FAT COCONUT MILK: These are usually sold in cartons, are much thinner, and often have a less distinct flavor than full-fat coconut milk. They are best used in flavors that can be turned into a sorbet, such as coconut or blackberry. If you do want a creamier taste with almond milk or reduced-fat coconut milk, you can simply add extra egg yolks.

HEAVY CREAM: This gives ice cream a more neutral flavor, along with a very thick and rich texture and taste. It goes well in heartier flavors such as Chocolate Ice Cream (page 16) and Holiday Spice Frozen Custard (page 129). Though cream is not paleo, it falls into Mark Sisson's "primal" category. (Sisson is a health and fitness author who runs the popular blog Mark's Daily Apple. He advocates a Primal diet, which is identical to the Paleo diet with the one exception—some dairy products are allowed.) Cream is also largely free of casein and lactose, two things that don't play nice with many people's bodies. Be sure to note that cream will turn into whipped cream if you spend more than a few seconds blending it at high speeds!

HALF AND HALF: Finally, half and half is what many store-bought ice cream cartons use as their base. I find it to be the most agreeable flavor and often use it when I want a "normal" ice cream taste or am making ice cream for friends and family. However, high-quality half and half is expensive and isn't paleo or primal, and many people can't tolerate it, so only use half and half if it works for your individual circumstance.

SWEETENERS

The second biggest way to change the flavor of your traditional ice cream recipes is to swap sweeteners. The sweetener won't change your ice cream's taste as much as the base will, but it definitely has an impact. The sweetener options are as follows:

HONEY: This is the most neutral-tasting nonrefined sweetener option. Any recipe in this book will go well with honey, though some work well with other sweeteners, too.

MAPLE SYRUP: This is another popular nonrefined sweetener used in many a paleo recipe. For me, maple syrup's taste is a bit too distinct to use in the average ice cream recipe. However, it does pair exceedingly well with certain flavors such as sweet potato (see recipe on page 74) and chocolate-covered bacon (see recipe on page 104). If you are a big maple syrup fan, feel free to substitute it in whenever you like.

COCONUT SUGAR: This is a sweetener that is halfway between honey and maple syrup. It does have a nonneutral flavor, but the taste of coconut sugar isn't overbearing. Coconut sugar can be used for most of the recipes in this book, especially if you are in the mood for a unique flavor of ice cream. Coconut sugar actually tastes a bit like maple syrup, so I personally always sub it in for the Canadian tree sap if maple syrup is called for.

LIQUID STEVIA: This is the least traditional sweetener option in this book. If you don't tolerate sugar or want to reduce your caloric intake, stevia is sugar-free and calorie-free. It will add sweetness to your ice cream, although some people don't like how stevia tastes. It tastes just fine to me, if not a bit simple and one-dimensional. The biggest difference between using liquid stevia and the other sweeteners is volume. You only need to use ¼ teaspoon of stevia for every ¼ cup of honey, maple syrup, or coconut sugar. Use extra egg yolks to make up for this lost volume and density.

CHANGING THE CONSISTENCY

EGG YOLKS: As suggested earlier, another way to tweak ice cream to your liking is by adjusting the number of egg yolks used. Using more egg yolks will result in a thicker, richer custard-style ice cream. Using less egg yolks will make your ice cream lighter and more of a sorbet. I will make a suggestion for egg yolk quantity in each recipe, but if you'd like your ice cream to be richer, you can add yolks; if you want your ice cream to be lighter, you can use fewer yolks.

XANTHAN GUM: The fourth and simplest way to modify these ice cream recipes is to add xanthan gum. This will allow your ice cream to keep overnight without getting icy. Many are scared by xanthan gum's name, thinking of it as some toxic additive. In reality, xanthan gum is simply a fermented carbohydrate. It has been shown to be more or less harmless in all human studies, though some people report mild intestinal distress. To be clear, xanthan gum is not a traditional paleo food, though experts such as Chris Kresser have declared it to be quite benign. If you try using xanthan gum and think it makes you feel a little funny, then only make as much ice cream as you and your companions will eat in one sitting or accept that your ice cream might get a little icy if left in the freezer.

***

Those are the four main ways to tweak each ice cream recipe to your liking, but the customization doesn't end there. If you make chocolate ice cream and find that it wasn't quite chocolaty enough for you, add more cocoa powder next time. You should experiment with your ice cream as much as possible so you can learn what works for you and what doesn't. When you know your own preferences, you can make a perfect batch every time!

INGREDIENT SUGGESTIONS

What follows is a list of ingredients required for the recipes in this book. If there is a particular variation of the ingredient that tastes best or is healthiest, I'll list it here.

COCONUT MILK: You can get either full-fat coconut milk, sold in cans, or reduced-fat coconut milk, sold in cartons. The practical differences between the two are described in the previous section. For both types, try to choose something with minimal ingredients you don't recognize on the back of the label. If you like to order online, I suggest buying the brand Native Forest, because its cans are BPA free.

ALMOND MILK: Make sure to check if your almond milk contains an added sweetener. If it does, adjust your own sweetener use appropriately. It is easiest to just buy unsweetened almond milk and use your own sweetener to jazz up the ice cream's flavor. As always, try to choose a product that minimizes the amount of unrecognizable ingredients on the back of the carton.

HALF AND HALF AND CREAM: The quality of half and half and cream varies a lot, so see if you can find a brand or farm you trust. Ideally, the cows that produce your dairy products would be pasture-raised, meaning they roam free on grassland instead of constantly being kept in a stall. If organic, pasture-raised dairy products are too costly, then just get regular half and half or cream. Your ice cream will still be healthier than what you get in the supermarket! Remember, though, that these dairy products aren't considered paleo, and many people don't digest them well. Only use half and half and cream if you are able to eat them without problems.

HONEY: Raw honey is the healthiest kind of honey around because its compounds aren't altered by the pasteurization process, so if you can afford it, that is ideal. If you can't find it in local stores or you find it to be too pricey at your farmer's market, then buying online is an option to check out. If you are on a budget, use whatever you can afford.

MAPLE SYRUP: Contrary to most people's intuition, Grade B maple syrup is the stuff you will want to use. It is less refined than its Grade A counterpart, so more nutrients are intact.

LIQUID STEVIA: Make sure to get pure liquid stevia, as it has less of an aftertaste than versions with extra additives.

EGGS: Eggs are healthiest when they come from hens that were allowed to roam free rather than hens kept in tight quarters. The labels to look for on an egg carton are "pasture-raised" and "organic." If these eggs are a bit out of your price range, settling for the much less regulated terms "free-range" and "cage-free" is your best bet.

XANTHAN GUM: The most widely available brand of xanthan gum is Bob's Red Mill. It is a cool, employee-owned company and makes a good product, so there is no need to look elsewhere. Remember, xanthan gum isn't considered paleo, though it has been shown to be fairly harmless in human studies.

CHOCOLATE: Because I am a proponent of homemade food, I suggest you try making your own chocolate. I've included a recipe for you to try if you are up for it. If not, don't worry, there is plenty of high-quality chocolate available for purchase in grocery stores. Try and get a bar with a cacao percentage of at least 60% to 70% for maximum nutritive value. If you prefer chocolate chips over broken-up chocolate bars, then go for those. Cacao nibs can also be used as a chocolate chip replacement and add a pleasant bitterness to your sweet ice cream.

COCOA POWDER: Make sure your cocoa powder is unsweetened so that you have full control over the sweetness of your final product. Also, the general rule for cocoa powder is the darker the color, the higher the quality.

FRUIT: Fresh, in-season fruit is the healthiest and tastiest option. If it is February, and you want some Blueberry Ice Cream (page 46), though, frozen fruit will have to do.

NUTS: Ideally, you'd soak and dehydrate all of your nuts. This reduces the amount of phytates and enzyme inhibitors, the natural defensive mechanisms present in your nuts. I am too lazy to do this, so I just make sure not to go too crazy on the nuts!

COCONUT: Your dried coconut can be flaked or shredded, but it should be unsweetened. You can find dried coconut in most stores, but I find prices to be best online.

COFFEE: As with most food, higher-quality coffee is more conducive to good health than cheap coffee. Beans roasted locally in small batches are at the top of the coffee pyramid, whereas big-brand coffee is generally of lesser quality. Having said that, the cost of some artisan coffees can be exorbitant and just isn't worth it for many of us. Just do what works for your individual situation and don't worry if your coffee isn't single origin, high-altitude, shade-grown, wet-processed, and organic!

EXTRACTS AND FLAVORINGS: Always go with real extracts over imitation flavorings. It can be tough sometimes to discern between the two, so read labels carefully.

FOOD QUALITY

Food quality is important. Using lower-quality ingredients not only impacts taste, but also can be detrimental to your health. Cream that comes from cows kept in stalls and fed cheap feed will have a different impact on your body than cream that comes from cows that spent their days grazing on green pastures. That being said, high-quality ingredients are often much more expensive. Pick your spots and do the best you can with the resources available to you.

SPICES: As with all foods on this list, fresh, organic spices are best. Spices lose their potency after two or three years, so if you haven't bought cinnamon in a few years, it is time to throw away your old stuff and get a new jar. If you just bought a new nonorganic jar a year ago, though, my advice would be to use it up to avoid wasting money. A good way to buy only as much spice as you need is to buy from the bulk section of your grocery store or supermarket.

TOOLS

ICE CREAM MACHINE: An ice cream machine is not necessary, but it is very, very helpful if you plan on making ice cream more than a few times per year. I bought mine on Craigslist, but you can also find reasonable prices on the Internet.

If you do not want to commit to buying an ice cream maker, you have two options:

1 **The slow option:** For this option you will have to create the ice cream mixture as per the instructions and then store the mixture in the freezer overnight. Using xanthan gum will be important here. If you can't wait overnight and don't want your ice cream to be as icy, then you can do the same as above but take the ice cream out and stir it well every thirty minutes. This process will take around three hours before your ice cream is ready to eat.

2 **The slightly labor-intensive option:** For this option you will also create the ice cream mixture as per the recipe's instructions, but this time you will put the mixture in a resealable plastic bag. This bag will go in the middle of another resealable bag, which will first be filled halfway with ice and ½ cup rock or kosher salt. Cover the outer bag with a towel or wear gloves and shake it up until the ice cream in the inner bag thickens. This should take twenty to thirty minutes.

TIME SAVER

If you're short on time, you can skip tempering the eggs and simply toss all of your ingredients in a blender and then freeze them in the ice cream maker. This saves quite a bit of time and effort, but you also open yourself up to the consumption of raw egg yolks, which poses the possible risk of salmonella. Do your research and make the best decision for yourself.

BLENDER: You'll use a blender to mix ingredients together and create a uniform-tasting ice cream. Very important to have for this book!

FOOD PROCESSOR: The food processor is only used to make Cookie Dough (page 156) and the banana- and cashew-based ice creams. A food processor isn't technically necessary for this cookbook, but it is quite helpful to have.

FINE-MESH STRAINER: These are used in the herb and spice recipes. Not completely necessary if you don't make those flavors.

CHAPTER 1: THE CLASSICS

In this chapter are the flavors we all remember and love from our childhoods. Simple, traditional—these flavors are probably what you thought of when you first picked up this book. Here they are: paleo versions of your favorite classic ice cream flavors.

CHOCOLATE ICE CREAM

This recipe does the childhood memories justice and allows you to get your chocolate fix! All of the sweeteners work well for this one, though honey will give you the most "normal" tasting chocolate. The flavor of coconut milk goes well with cocoa powder, though cream is great, too, if you want a very thick chocolate ice cream. I recommend topping it with a decadent berry sauce, such as the Strawberry Sauce (page 153).

YIELD: About ¾ quart

1 (13.5-ounce) can coconut milk

4 tablespoons honey

¼ teaspoon xanthan gum (optional)

3 tablespoons cocoa powder

1 teaspoon vanilla extract

½ teaspoon salt

3 egg yolks

1   In a medium saucepan over low heat, combine coconut milk, honey, xanthan gum (if using), cocoa powder, vanilla extract, and salt. Stir continuously until the mixture thickens enough to coat the back of a spoon, about 8 minutes. Set aside.

2   In a heat-safe bowl, whisk the egg yolks until they reach a fluffy consistency. Add a small ladle of the warm mixture and stir until combined. Continue adding the warm mixture, one ladle at a time, until it's completely mixed into the egg yolks. Don't add too much of the warm mixture at once or you may end up with scrambled eggs!

3   Cover the mixture and refrigerate until completely chilled (about 8 hours or up to 2 days).

4   Freeze the mixture in your ice cream maker according to the manufacturer's instructions and enjoy! If you don't plan on serving the ice cream immediately, transfer to a freezer-proof container and freeze up to 1 week (or 2 months if you use xanthan gum and place

a layer of plastic wrap on the surface of the ice cream). To serve, remove from freezer and let sit about 15 minutes, or until desired texture is reached.

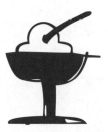

STRAWBERRY ICE CREAM

To preserve maximum sweetness of the strawberries, wipe them with a damp paper towel rather than washing all at once. Also, if you want to mix up the classic strawberry flavor, you can add a shot of brandy or the juice of one lemon to the mixture.

YIELD: About 1 quart

1 (13.5-ounce) can coconut milk

3 tablespoons honey

¼ teaspoon xanthan gum (optional)

4 egg yolks

2 cups fresh strawberries, hulled

1 In a medium saucepan over low heat, combine coconut milk, honey, and xanthan gum (if using). Stir continuously until the mixture thickens enough to coat the back of a spoon, about 8 minutes. Set aside.

2 In a heat-safe bowl, whisk the egg yolks until they reach a fluffy consistency. Add a small ladle of the warm mixture and stir until combined. Continue adding the warm mixture, one ladle at a time, until it's completely mixed into the egg yolks. Don't add too much of the warm mixture at once or you may end up with scrambled eggs!

3 Cover the mixture and refrigerate until completely chilled (about 8 hours or up to 2 days).

4 Blend chilled mixture and strawberries in a blender until smooth, about 30 seconds. Or, alternatively, if you like small strawberry chunks in your ice cream, you can blend to personal preference.

5 Freeze the mixture in your ice cream maker according to the manufacturer's instructions. If you aren't serving the ice cream immediately, transfer to a freezer-proof container and freeze up to 1 week (or 2 months if you use xanthan gum and place a layer of plastic wrap on the surface of the ice cream). To serve, remove from freezer and let sit 15 minutes, or until desired texture is reached.

VANILLA ICE CREAM

Vanilla is the only ice cream flavor I ate growing up, and I still enjoy a good bowl of vanilla every now and then. If you are using coconut milk as the base, as with many of these recipes, I recommend using slightly more vanilla extract to stand out against the coconut.

YIELD: About ¾ quart

1 (13.5-ounce) can coconut milk

3 tablespoons honey

¼ teaspoon xanthan gum (optional)

3 teaspoons vanilla extract or 1 vanilla bean pod

3 egg yolks

1 In a medium saucepan over low heat, combine coconut milk, honey, xanthan gum (if using), and vanilla. If you are using a vanilla bean, split it in half lengthwise and scrape the seeds into the creamy mixture. Stir continuously until the mixture thickens enough to coat the back of a spoon, about 8 minutes. Set aside.

2 In a heat-safe bowl, whisk the egg yolks until they reach a fluffy consistency. Add a small ladle of the warm mixture and stir until combined. Continue adding the warm mixture, one ladle at a time, until it's completely mixed into the egg yolks. Don't add too much of the warm mixture at once or you may end up with scrambled eggs!

3 Cover the mixture and refrigerate until completely chilled (about 8 hours or up to 2 days).

4 Freeze the mixture in your ice cream maker according to the manufacturer's instructions and enjoy! If you don't plan on serving the ice cream immediately, transfer to a freezer-proof container and freeze up to 1 week (or 2 months if you use xanthan gum and place a layer of plastic wrap on the surface of the ice cream). To serve, remove from freezer and let sit about 15 minutes, or until desired texture is reached.

BUTTER PECAN ICE CREAM

Life is always better with butter! That's my motto, anyway, and I try to live it out. Adding butter to my coffee (try it!) is one way I do this, and butter pecan ice cream is another.

YIELD: About 1 quart

1 (13.5-ounce) can coconut milk

4 tablespoons honey

¼ teaspoon xanthan gum (optional)

6 tablespoons butter

1 teaspoon vanilla extract

2 egg yolks

1½ cups coarsely chopped pecans

1 In a medium saucepan over low heat, combine coconut milk, honey, xanthan gum (if using), butter, and vanilla extract. Stir continuously until the mixture thickens enough to coat the back of a spoon, about 8 minutes. Set aside.

2 In a heat-safe bowl, whisk the egg yolks until they reach a fluffy consistency. Add a small ladle of the warm mixture and stir until combined. Continue adding the warm mixture, one ladle at a time, until it's completely mixed into the egg yolks. Don't add too much of the warm mixture at once or you may end up with scrambled eggs!

3 Cover the mixture and refrigerate until completely chilled (about 8 hours or up to 2 days).

4 Freeze the mixture in your ice cream maker according to the manufacturer's instructions.

5 Sprinkle in pecans just as your ice cream finishes hardening and enjoy! If you don't plan on serving the ice cream immediately, transfer to a freezer-proof container and freeze up to 1 week (or 2 months if you use xanthan gum and place a layer of plastic wrap on the surface of the ice cream). To serve, remove from freezer and let sit about 15 minutes, or until desired texture is reached.

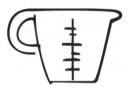

COOKIE DOUGH ICE CREAM

Ahh, cookies, another much maligned food in the paleosphere. Many paleo eaters refer to them as candy cigarettes and employ a strict no-cookie policy. If you love cookies, here is your paleo answer. For this recipe, you can take a cue from Ben and Jerry's and "half-bake" your Cookie Dough balls by putting them on a greased baking sheet and baking them in the oven at 350°F for 5 minutes.

YIELD: About 1 quart

1 (13.5-ounce) can coconut milk

3 tablespoons honey

¼ teaspoon xanthan gum (optional)

2 teaspoons vanilla extract or 1 vanilla bean

3 egg yolks

8 ½-inch Cookie Dough balls (page 156)

1 In a medium saucepan over low heat, combine coconut milk, honey, xanthan gum (if using), and vanilla. If you are using a vanilla bean, split it in half lengthwise and scrape the seeds into the creamy mixture. Stir continuously until the mixture thickens enough to coat the back of a spoon, about 8 minutes. Set aside.

2 In a heat-safe bowl, whisk the egg yolks until they reach a fluffy consistency. Add a small ladle of the warm mixture and stir until combined. Continue adding the warm mixture, one ladle at a time, until it's completely mixed into the egg yolks. Don't add too much of the warm mixture at once or you may end up with scrambled eggs!

3 Cover the mixture and refrigerate until completely chilled (about 8 hours or up to 2 days).

4 Freeze the mixture in your ice cream maker according to the manufacturer's instructions.

5 Drop in Cookie Dough balls just as your ice cream reaches your desired consistency and enjoy! If you don't plan on serving the ice cream immediately, transfer to a freezer-proof container and freeze up to 1 week (or 2 months if you use xanthan gum and place a layer of plastic wrap on the surface of the ice cream). To serve, remove from freezer and let sit about 15 minutes, or until desired texture is reached.

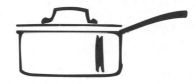

MINT CHOCOLATE CHIP ICE CREAM

If using the homemade Chocolate Pieces recipe (page 148) described in the introduction, make sure it is very frozen before adding. Using homemade chocolate will make this flavor taste very sophisticated, which makes it a good one if you want to impress someone with your gourmet cooking.

YIELD: About ¾ quart

1 (13.5-ounce) can coconut milk

4 tablespoons honey

¼ teaspoon xanthan gum (optional)

1 teaspoon peppermint extract

3 egg yolks

⅓ cup dark chocolate chips or Chocolate Pieces (page 148)

1 In a medium saucepan over low heat, combine coconut milk, honey, xanthan gum (if using), and peppermint extract. Stir continuously until the mixture thickens enough to coat the back of a spoon, about 8 minutes. Set aside.

2 In a heat-safe bowl, whisk the egg yolks until they reach a fluffy consistency. Add a small ladle of the warm mixture and stir until combined. Continue adding the warm mixture, one ladle at a time, until it's completely mixed into the egg yolks. Don't add too much of the warm mixture at once or you may end up with scrambled eggs!

3 Cover the mixture and refrigerate until completely chilled (about 8 hours or up to 2 days).

4 Freeze the mixture in your ice cream maker according to the manufacturer's instructions.

5 Fold in chocolate chips just as your ice cream starts to reach your desired consistency. If you don't plan on serving the ice cream

immediately, transfer to a freezer-proof container and freeze up to 1 week (or 2 months if you use xanthan gum and place a layer of plastic wrap on the surface of the ice cream). To serve, remove from freezer and let sit about 15 minutes, or until desired texture is reached.

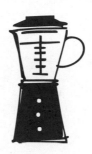

RUM RAISIN ICE CREAM

This classic flavor seems to have fallen by the wayside in recent years, but with this recipe I can foresee a comeback. If you invite a few friends over, make some mixed drinks with rum and drink them while the ice cream freezes. I suggest equal parts dark rum, coconut rum, and pineapple juice, a favorite of Kelsey's parents, Pat and Trisha.

YIELD: About ¾ quart

1 (13.5-ounce) can coconut milk

4 tablespoons honey

¼ teaspoon xanthan gum (optional)

2 teaspoons vanilla extract

3 egg yolks

3 tablespoons of dark rum

¼ cup raisins

1 In a medium saucepan over low heat, combine coconut milk, honey, xanthan gum (if using), and vanilla extract. Stir continuously until the mixture thickens enough to coat the back of a spoon, about 8 minutes. Set aside.

2 In a heat-safe bowl, whisk the egg yolks until they reach a fluffy consistency. Add a small ladle of the warm mixture and stir until combined. Continue adding the warm mixture, one ladle at a time, until it's completely mixed into the egg yolks. Don't add too much of the warm mixture at once or you may end up with scrambled eggs!

3 Mix in rum.

4 Cover the mixture and refrigerate until completely chilled (about 8 hours or up to 2 days).

5 Freeze the mixture in your ice cream maker according to the manufacturer's instructions.

6 Sprinkle in raisins just as your ice cream finishes hardening and enjoy! If you don't plan on serving the ice cream immediately, transfer to a freezer-proof container and freeze up to 1 week (or 2 months if you use xanthan gum and place a layer of plastic wrap on the surface of the ice cream). To serve, remove from freezer and let sit about 15 minutes, or until desired texture is reached.

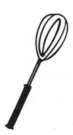

ORANGE SHERBET

Remember Vanilla and Orange Sherbet Dixie Cups? If you want to recreate that flavor combo, then make orange cream ice cream in the morning, freeze it, make vanilla ice cream after dinner, and combine for dessert.

Using cream in this recipe makes for a particularly rich orange cream flavor, and using almond milk will produce a lighter-tasting sherbet.

YIELD: About 1 quart

1 (13.5-ounce) can coconut milk

4 tablespoons honey

¼ teaspoon xanthan gum (optional)

1½ cups freshly squeezed orange juice

1 tablespoon fresh lemon juice

1 teaspoon vanilla extract

4 egg yolks

1 tablespoon orange zest

1   In a medium saucepan over low heat, combine coconut milk, honey, xanthan gum (if using), orange juice, lemon juice, and vanilla extract. Stir continuously until the mixture thickens enough to coat the back of a spoon, about 8 minutes. Set aside.

2   In a heat-safe bowl, whisk the egg yolks until they reach a fluffy consistency. Add a small ladle of the warm mixture and stir until combined. Continue adding the warm mixture, one ladle at a time, until it's completely mixed into the egg yolks. Don't add too much of the warm mixture at once or you may end up with scrambled eggs!

3   Cover the mixture and refrigerate until completely chilled (about 8 hours or up to 2 days).

4   Mix in orange zest.

5 Freeze the mixture in your ice cream maker according to the manufacturer's instructions and enjoy! If you don't plan on serving the ice cream immediately, transfer to a freezer-proof container and freeze up to 1 week (or 2 months if you use xanthan gum and place a layer of plastic wrap on the surface of the ice cream). To serve, remove from freezer and let sit about 15 minutes, or until desired texture is reached.

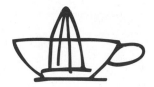

FRESH TRACKS ICE CREAM

This flavor is a fresh take on the classic Moose Tracks ice cream flavor. Coincidentally, the rich chocolate and almond butter combination works quite well after a long day at the slopes. I personally enjoy the texture of "chunky" almond butter in this one, though you can get the same effect by adding in ¼ cup of toasted almond slivers.

YIELD: About ¾ quart

1 (13.5-ounce) can coconut milk

4 tablespoons honey

¼ teaspoon xanthan gum (optional)

4 egg yolks

2 teaspoons vanilla extract

¼ cup almond butter

⅛ cup Chocolate Pieces (page 148)

⅛ cup Chocolate Sauce (page 149)

1 In a medium saucepan over low heat, combine coconut milk, honey, and xanthan gum (if using). Stir continuously until the mixture thickens enough to coat the back of a spoon, about 8 minutes. Set aside.

2 In a heat-safe bowl, whisk the egg yolks until they reach a fluffy consistency. Add a small ladle of the warm mixture and stir until combined. Continue adding the warm mixture, one ladle at a time, until it's completely mixed into the egg yolks. Don't add too much of the warm mixture at once or you may end up with scrambled eggs!

3 Cover the mixture and refrigerate until completely chilled (about 8 hours or up to 2 days).

4 In a blender, combine chilled mixture with vanilla extract and almond butter and blend for 30 seconds.

5 Freeze the mixture in your ice cream maker according to the manufacturer's instructions.

6 Mix in Chocolate Pieces and Chocolate Sauce when ice cream is nearly finished and enjoy! If you don't plan on serving the ice cream immediately, transfer to a freezer-proof container and freeze up to 1 week (or 2 months if you use xanthan gum and place a layer of plastic wrap on the surface of the ice cream). To serve, remove from freezer and let sit about 15 minutes, or until desired texture is reached.

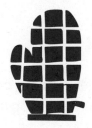

MOCHA CHIP ICE CREAM

You top this flavor with coffee grounds for additional texture and taste. If you are sensitive to chocolate flavor, then you can omit the cocoa powder and still enjoy coffee ice cream with homemade Chocolate Pieces.

YIELD: About ¾ quart

1 (13.5-ounce) can coconut milk

4 tablespoons honey

¼ teaspoon xanthan gum (optional)

2 tablespoons cocoa powder

1 shot of espresso or 1½ cups coarsely ground coffee beans

3 egg yolks

½ cup Chocolate Pieces (page 148)

1 In a medium saucepan over low heat, combine coconut milk, honey, xanthan gum (if using), and cocoa powder.

2 Add the shot of espresso, or if using coffee grounds, add beans and let simmer on low until the mixture reaches a deep brown. Once steeped (about 10 minutes), strain with a fine-mesh strainer to remove coffee grounds. Stir continuously until the mixture thickens enough to coat the back of a spoon, about 8 minutes. Set aside.

3 In a heat-safe bowl, whisk the egg yolks until they reach a fluffy consistency. Add a small ladle of the warm mixture and stir until combined. Continue adding the warm mixture, one ladle at a time, until it's completely mixed into the egg yolks. Don't add too much of the warm mixture at once or you may end up with scrambled eggs!

4 Cover the mixture and refrigerate until completely chilled (about 8 hours or up to 2 days).

5 Freeze the mixture in your ice cream maker according to the manufacturer's instructions.

6 Sprinkle in Chocolate Pieces just as your ice cream finishes hardening and enjoy! If you don't plan on serving the ice cream immediately, transfer to a freezer-proof container and freeze up to 1 week (or 2 months if you use xanthan gum and place a layer of plastic wrap on the surface of the ice cream). To serve, remove from freezer and let sit about 15 minutes, or until desired texture is reached.

CHOCOLATE CHIP ICE CREAM

Chocolate chip is a good flavor for those times when vanilla is too simple, but chocolate is too rich. Why not compromise and put pieces of homemade chocolate in your ice cream? If you prefer real chocolate chips, feel free to use them. I won't be offended!

YIELD: About ¾ quart

1 (13.5-ounce) can coconut milk

3 tablespoons honey

¼ teaspoon xanthan gum (optional)

2 teaspoons vanilla extract

3 egg yolks

¼ cup Chocolate Pieces (page 148)

1 In a medium saucepan over low heat, combine coconut milk, honey, xanthan gum (if using), and vanilla extract. Stir continuously until the mixture thickens enough to coat the back of a spoon, about 8 minutes. Set aside.

2 In a heat-safe bowl, whisk the egg yolks until they reach a fluffy consistency. Add a small ladle of the warm mixture and stir until combined. Continue adding the warm mixture, one ladle at a time, until it's completely mixed into the egg yolks. Don't add too much of the warm mixture at once or you may end up with scrambled eggs!

3 Cover the mixture and refrigerate until completely chilled (about 8 hours or up to 2 days).

4 Freeze the mixture in your ice cream maker according to the manufacturer's instructions.

5   Mix in Chocolate Pieces when ice cream is nearly finished and enjoy! If you don't plan on serving the ice cream immediately, transfer to a freezer-proof container and freeze up to 1 week (or 2 months if you use xanthan gum and place a layer of plastic wrap on the surface of the ice cream). To serve, remove from freezer and let sit about 15 minutes, or until desired texture is reached.

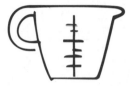

CHAPTER 2: FUN AND FRUITY

Fruit-flavored ice cream is awesome. But fruit-flavored ice cream using fresh fruit is much, much better. I think that is one of the main areas where homemade ice cream trumps store-bought stuff by a wide margin. Even if you are using frozen fruit, it was likely frozen fresh at peak ripeness. Using fresh or frozen fruit is much healthier and tastier than the syrups and other fake flavorings used in store-bought ice cream!

CHERRY CHOCOLATE ICE CREAM

I am usually not a fan of cherry-flavored sweets, but this cherry ice cream is to die for! I suspect it is because this ice cream tastes like actual cherries. Cherry ice cream is especially good with homemade dark chocolate, though of course it can be omitted if you want a pure cherry flavor.

YIELD: About 1 quart

1 (13.5-ounce) can coconut milk

4 tablespoons honey

¼ teaspoon xanthan gum (optional)

4 egg yolks

2 cups fresh cherries, pitted

½ cup Shaved Chocolate (page 148)

1 In a medium saucepan over low heat, combine coconut milk, honey, and xanthan gum (if using). Stir continuously until the mixture thickens enough to coat the back of a spoon, about 8 minutes. Set aside.

2 In a heat-safe bowl, whisk the egg yolks until they reach a fluffy consistency. Add a small ladle of the warm mixture and stir until combined. Continue adding the warm mixture, one ladle at a time, until it's completely mixed into the egg yolks. Don't add too much of the warm mixture at once or you may end up with scrambled eggs!

3 Cover the mixture and refrigerate until completely chilled (about 8 hours or up to 2 days).

4 Blend chilled mixture and cherries in a blender until smooth, about 30 seconds. Or, alternatively, if you like small cherry chunks in your ice cream, you can blend to personal preference.

5   Freeze the mixture in your ice cream maker according to the manufacturer's instructions.

6   Sprinkle in chocolate shavings just as your ice cream reaches your desired consistency and enjoy! If you don't plan on serving the ice cream immediately, transfer to a freezer-proof container and freeze up to 1 week (or 2 months if using xanthan gum and place a layer of plastic wrap on the surface of the ice cream). To serve, remove from freezer and let sit about 15 minutes, or until desired texture is reached.

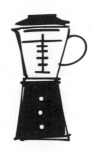

COCONUT ICE CREAM

Obviously, this is the perfect recipe to use coconut milk. The shredded coconut adds a fun and unique texture, and you can make it work even better as an aesthetically pleasing garnish if you toast it first.

YIELD: About ¾ quart

1 (13.5-ounce) can coconut milk

4 tablespoons honey

¼ teaspoon xanthan gum (optional)

1 cup coconut cream

4 egg yolks

2 tablespoons unsweetened shredded coconut flakes

1 In a medium saucepan over low heat, combine coconut milk, honey, xanthan gum (if using), and coconut cream. Stir continuously until the mixture thickens enough to coat the back of a spoon, about 8 minutes. Set aside.

2 In a heat-safe bowl, whisk the egg yolks until they reach a fluffy consistency. Add a small ladle of the warm mixture and stir until combined. Continue adding the warm mixture, one ladle at a time, until it's completely mixed into the egg yolks. Don't add too much of the warm mixture at once or you may end up with scrambled eggs!

3 Cover the mixture and refrigerate until completely chilled (about 8 hours or up to 2 days).

4 Toast the coconut flakes if desired. Spread out evenly on a baking sheet and toast at 350°F for 3–5 minutes, keeping an eye out so that they don't burn. You can take the coconut flakes out of the oven and redistribute them if you want them to be evenly toasted. Let cool completely. Mix in shredded coconut flakes.

5 Freeze the mixture in your ice cream maker according to the manufacturer's instructions and enjoy! If you don't plan on serving

the ice cream immediately, transfer to a freezer-proof container and freeze up to 1 week (or 2 months if you use xanthan gum and place a layer of plastic wrap on the surface of the ice cream). To serve, remove from freezer and let sit about 15 minutes, or until desired texture is reached.

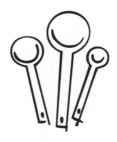

AVOCADO BANANA ICE CREAM

The avocado adds an impressive amount of creaminess to this ice cream while also adding some nutritional oomph. If you don't like how avocados taste, don't rule this flavor out, because the taste of banana definitely takes center stage. If you end up loving this one, make sure to try the banana-based recipes later in the book.

YIELD: About 1 ¼ quarts

1 (13.5-ounce) can coconut milk

2 tablespoons honey

¼ teaspoon xanthan gum (optional)

2 egg yolks

4 ripe bananas

1 ripe medium-sized avocado

1 In a medium saucepan over low heat, combine coconut milk, honey, and xanthan gum, if using. Stir continuously until the mixture thickens enough to coat the back of a spoon, about 8 minutes. Set aside.

2 In a heat-safe bowl, whisk the egg yolks until they reach a fluffy consistency. Add a small ladle of the warm mixture and stir until combined. Continue adding the warm mixture, one ladle at a time, until it's completely mixed into the egg yolks. Don't add too much of the warm mixture at once or you may end up with scrambled eggs!

3 Cover the mixture and refrigerate until completely chilled (about 8 hours or up to 2 days).

4 Blend chilled mixture with bananas and avocado in a blender until smooth, about 30 seconds.

5 Freeze the mixture in your ice cream maker according to the manufacturer's instructions and enjoy! If you don't plan on serving

the ice cream immediately, transfer to a freezer-proof container and freeze up to 1 week (or 2 months if you use xanthan gum and place a layer of plastic wrap on the surface of the ice cream). To serve, remove from freezer and let sit about 15 minutes, or until desired texture is reached.

BANANA WALNUT ICE CREAM

Bananas and walnuts pair together well, especially in ice cream. If you want to take this recipe to the next level, try toasting your walnuts. If you really want to take this recipe to the next level, try candying your walnuts in coconut sugar. Pecans work well, too, if that is more your style.

YIELD: About 1¼ quarts

1 (13.5-ounce) can coconut milk

2 tablespoons honey

¼ teaspoon xanthan gum (optional)

4 egg yolks

¼ teaspoon salt

4 ripe bananas

1 cup walnuts, coarsely chopped

1 In a medium saucepan over low heat, combine coconut milk, honey, and xanthan gum (if using). Stir continuously until the mixture thickens enough to coat the back of a spoon, about 8 minutes. Set aside.

2 In a heat-safe bowl, whisk the egg yolks until they reach a fluffy consistency. Add a small ladle of the warm mixture and stir until combined. Continue adding the warm mixture, one ladle at a time, until it's completely mixed into the egg yolks. Don't add too much of the warm mixture at once or you may end up with scrambled eggs!

3 Cover the mixture and refrigerate until completely chilled (about 8 hours or up to 2 days).

4 To toast the walnuts, spread evenly in a single layer on a baking sheet and cook at 350°F for 8–10 minutes, turning after five minutes. Let cool completely.

4   Blend chilled mixture with salt and bananas in a blender on high until smooth.

5   Freeze the mixture in your ice cream maker according to the manufacturer's instructions.

6   Stir in walnuts and enjoy! If you don't plan on serving the ice cream immediately, transfer to a freezer-proof container and freeze up to 1 week (or 2 months if you use xanthan gum and place a layer of plastic wrap on the surface of the ice cream). To serve, remove from freezer and let sit about 15 minutes, or until desired texture is reached.

CANDIED WALNUTS

It is easy to candy walnuts! Just mix 1 cup of walnuts with ⅓ cup coconut sugar in a medium saucepan and cook over medium heat. Stir continuously and remove the mixture from heat after the walnuts are coated in melted coconut sugar, about five minutes. Pour the candied walnuts onto a sheet of parchment paper and allow them to cool completely.

BLUEBERRY ICE CREAM

Not only do blueberries turn your ice cream an awesome shade of purple, they also pack a serious nutritional punch. Quite the win-win situation!

YIELD: About 1 quart

1 (13.5-ounce) can coconut milk

3 tablespoons honey

¼ teaspoon xanthan gum (optional)

4 egg yolks

2 cups fresh blueberries

1 In a medium saucepan over low heat, combine coconut milk, honey, and xanthan gum (if using). Stir continuously until the mixture thickens enough to coat the back of a spoon, about 8 minutes. Set aside.

2 In a heat-safe bowl, whisk the egg yolks until they reach a fluffy consistency. Add a small ladle of the warm mixture and stir until combined. Continue adding the warm mixture, one ladle at a time, until it's completely mixed into the egg yolks. Don't add too much of the warm mixture at once or you may end up with scrambled eggs!

3 Cover the mixture and refrigerate until completely chilled (about 8 hours or up to 2 days).

4 Blend chilled mixture and blueberries in a blender until smooth, about 30 seconds.

5 Freeze the mixture in your ice cream maker according to the manufacturer's instructions and enjoy! If you don't plan on serving the ice cream immediately, transfer to a freezer-proof container and freeze up to 1 week (or 2 months if you use xanthan gum and place a layer of plastic wrap on the surface of the ice cream). To serve, remove from freezer and let sit about 15 minutes, or until desired texture is reached.

CHERRY VANILLA ICE CREAM

A popular drink some of my friends would have when I was growing up was Cherry Vanilla Coke. I can see why after combining vanilla extract and fresh cherries for this recipe! Raspberries work well in the place of cherries, too, if that combination sounds more appealing.

YIELD: About 1 quart

1 (13.5-ounce) can coconut milk

4 tablespoons honey

¼ teaspoon xanthan gum (optional)

4 egg yolks

2 cups fresh cherries, pitted

3 teaspoons vanilla extract

1 In a medium saucepan over low heat, combine coconut milk, honey, and xanthan gum (if using). Stir continuously until the mixture thickens enough to coat the back of a spoon, about 8 minutes. Set aside.

2 In a heat-safe bowl, whisk the egg yolks until they reach a fluffy consistency. Add a small ladle of the warm mixture and stir until combined. Continue adding the warm mixture, one ladle at a time, until it's completely mixed into the egg yolks. Don't add too much of the warm mixture at once or you may end up with scrambled eggs!

3 Cover the mixture and refrigerate until completely chilled (about 8 hours or up to 2 days).

4 Blend chilled mixture, cherries, and vanilla extract in a blender until smooth, about 30 seconds. Or, alternatively, if you like small cherry chunks in your ice cream, you can blend to personal preference.

5 Freeze the mixture in your ice cream maker according to the manufacturer's instructions and enjoy! If you don't plan on serving the ice cream immediately, transfer to a freezer-proof container and freeze up to 1 week (or 2 months if you use xanthan gum and place a layer of plastic wrap on the surface of the ice cream). To serve, remove from freezer and let sit about 15 minutes, or until desired texture is reached.

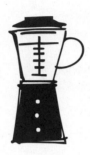

CHOCOLATE RASPBERRY SWIRL ICE CREAM

The combination of raspberries and chocolate is fantastic. This recipe can be made as written or to leave out the raspberry puree and pour it on as a topping after the chocolate ice cream is done and scooped. Either way, you will get your much-needed raspberry chocolate fix.

YIELD: About ¾ quart

1 (13.5-ounce) can coconut milk

4 tablespoons honey

¼ teaspoon xanthan gum (optional)

4 egg yolks

2 tablespoons cocoa powder

¼ teaspoon vanilla extract

⅔ cup raspberries

1 In a medium saucepan over low heat, combine coconut milk, honey, and xanthan gum (if using). Stir continuously until the mixture thickens enough to coat the back of a spoon, about 8 minutes. Set aside.

2 In a heat-safe bowl, whisk the egg yolks until they reach a fluffy consistency. Add a small ladle of the warm mixture and stir until combined. Continue adding the warm mixture, one ladle at a time, until it's completely mixed into the egg yolks. Don't add too much of the warm mixture at once or you may end up with scrambled eggs!

3 Cover the mixture and refrigerate until completely chilled (about 8 hours or up to 2 days).

4 Blend chilled mixture with cocoa powder and vanilla extract in a blender until a homogeneous texture is achieved, about 15 seconds.

5 Freeze the mixture in your ice cream maker according to the manufacturer's instructions.

6 While ice cream is thickening, mash raspberries with a fork or blender until they become more of a puree than fruit.

7 As the ice cream starts to harden, pour the raspberry puree into the ice cream maker. Enjoy! If you don't plan on serving the ice cream immediately, transfer to a freezer-proof container and freeze up to 1 week (or 2 months if you use xanthan gum and place a layer of plastic wrap on the surface of the ice cream). To serve, remove from freezer and let sit about 15 minutes, or until desired texture is reached.

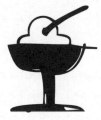

CHAPTER 3: FROZEN "DRINKS"

One of my favorite parts of cooking is combining foods in nontraditional ways. One way I do this is by keeping the flavor of the food but changing its medium. In this case, I had a great time translating some of my favorite drinks into ice cream flavors. Bottoms up!

STRAWBERRY BANANA ICE CREAM

Strawberry banana works in smoothies, so why not in ice cream? This is a very refreshing flavor that can bring you back to summer any day of the year thanks to frozen strawberries. If there are other flavor combinations you love in smoothies, you should definitely try them out in ice cream form, too!

YIELD: About 1 quart

1 (13.5-ounce) can coconut milk

2 tablespoons honey

¼ teaspoon xanthan gum (optional)

4 egg yolks

2 ripe bananas

1½ cups fresh strawberries, hulled

1   In a medium saucepan over low heat, combine coconut milk, honey, and xanthan gum (if using). Stir continuously until the mixture thickens enough to coat the back of a spoon, about 8 minutes. Set aside.

2   In a heat-safe bowl, whisk the egg yolks until they reach a fluffy consistency. Add a small ladle of the warm mixture and stir until combined. Continue adding the warm mixture, one ladle at a time, until it's completely mixed into the egg yolks. Don't add too much of the warm mixture at once or you may end up with scrambled eggs!

3   Cover the mixture and refrigerate until completely chilled (about 8 hours or up to 2 days).

4   Blend chilled mixture, strawberries, and bananas in a blender until smooth, about 30 seconds.

5   Freeze the mixture in your ice cream maker according to the manufacturer's instructions and enjoy! If you don't plan on serving

the ice cream immediately, transfer to a freezer-proof container and freeze up to 1 week (or 2 months if you use xanthan gum and place a layer of plastic wrap on the surface of the ice cream). To serve, remove from freezer and let sit about 15 minutes, or until desired texture is reached.

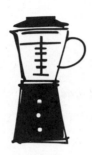

CHAI TEA ICE CREAM

This was the flavor that started it all! Every time I eat it, I think back to that wonderful picnic in the Washington Park Arboretum. Ahhh, the memories! If you want to continue the tradition, scoop your Chai Tea Ice Cream in an airtight container and stick it in the freezer. Then, when it is time to head out to your chosen spot of grassy earth, put it on some ice in a small cooler. Spaghetti squash and kale salad optional!

YIELD: About ¾ quart

1 (13.5-ounce) can coconut milk

3 tablespoons honey

¼ teaspoon xanthan gum (optional)

5 tablespoons full-bodied black tea

1 star anise

10 whole cloves

10 whole allspices

2 cinnamon sticks

10 whole white peppercorns

5 cardamom pods, opened to seeds

1 2-inch piece fresh ginger

3 egg yolks

1 In a medium saucepan over low heat, combine coconut milk, honey, xanthan gum (if using), tea, and all spices. Let simmer until the mixture turns an earthy brown, stirring occasionally, about 45 minutes. Set aside.

2 Strain mixture using a fine-mesh strainer.

3 In a heat-safe bowl, whisk the egg yolks until they reach a fluffy consistency. Add a small ladle of the warm mixture and stir until combined. Continue adding the warm mixture, one ladle at a time, until it's completely mixed into the egg yolks. Don't add too much of the warm mixture at once or you may end up with scrambled eggs!

4 Cover the mixture and refrigerate until completely chilled (about 8 hours or up to 2 days).

5 Freeze the mixture in your ice cream maker according to the manufacturer's instructions and enjoy! If you don't plan on serving the ice cream immediately, transfer to a freezer-proof container and freeze up to 1 week (or 2 months if you use xanthan gum and place a layer of plastic wrap on the surface of the ice cream). To serve, remove from freezer and let sit about 15 minutes, or until desired texture is reached.

ESPRESSO ICE CREAM

My mom loves coffee ice cream, and I have to say that I inherited the coffee-loving gene. Though some might not like it, I also enjoy sprinkling some coffee grounds into this recipe after it finishes freezing. They add a funky texture and give the flavor another layer. For a vanilla latte effect, add 2 teaspoons of vanilla extract.

YIELD: About ¾ quart

1 (13.5-ounce) can coconut milk

4 tablespoons honey

¼ teaspoon xanthan gum (optional)

1 shot of espresso or 1½ cups ground coffee beans

3 egg yolks

1 In a medium saucepan over low heat, combine coconut milk, honey, and xanthan gum (if using).

2 Add the shot of espresso, or if using coffee grounds, add beans and let simmer on low until the mixture reaches a deep brown, about 10 minutes. Once steeped, strain the mixture with a fine-mesh strainer to remove grounds. Set aside.

3 In a heat-safe bowl, whisk the egg yolks until they reach a fluffy consistency. Add a small ladle of the warm mixture and stir until combined. Continue adding the warm mixture, one ladle at a time, until it's completely mixed into the egg yolks. Don't add too much of the warm mixture at once or you may end up with scrambled eggs!

4 Cover the mixture and refrigerate until completely chilled (about 8 hours or up to 2 days).

5 Freeze the mixture in your ice cream maker according to the manufacturer's instructions and enjoy!

GREEN TEA ICE CREAM

Though tea bags work pretty well, I recommend using matcha powder to save on time and produce a more powerful flavor. Green tea is one of those things that I have always wanted to get into drinking because of its health-enhancing properties, but I never particularly liked the taste. I figure green tea ice cream is a good way to gradually adjust to the flavor.

YIELD: About ¾ quart

1 (13.5-ounce) can coconut milk

4 tablespoons honey

¼ teaspoon xanthan gum (optional)

1 tablespoon matcha tea powder or ½ cup loose green tea or 8 green tea bags

3 egg yolks

1 In a medium saucepan over low heat, combine coconut milk, honey, and xanthan gum (if using).

2 Add green tea powder. Or, if using loose green tea leaves or bags, add tea and let simmer on low heat until the ice cream reaches a dark cream color, stirring occasionally. Once steeped, about 30 minutes, strain the warm mixture with a fine-mesh strainer, to remove leaves or tea bags. Set aside.

3 In a heat-safe bowl, whisk the egg yolks until they reach a fluffy consistency. Add a small ladle of the warm mixture and stir until combined. Continue adding the warm mixture, one ladle at a time, until it's completely mixed into the egg yolks. Don't add too much of the warm mixture at once or you may end up with scrambled eggs!

4 Cover the mixture and refrigerate until completely chilled (about 8 hours or up to 2 days).

5 Freeze the mixture in your ice cream maker according to the manufacturer's instructions and enjoy! If you don't plan on serving

the ice cream immediately, transfer to a freezer-proof container and freeze up to 1 week (or 2 months if you use xanthan gum and place a layer of plastic wrap on the surface of the ice cream). To serve, remove from freezer and let sit about 15 minutes, or until desired texture is reached.

WHITE RUSSIAN ICE CREAM

For the full White Russian effect, you can try using cream or half and half instead of coconut milk if you tolerate dairy. If, like my grandma, you are a member of chocoholics anonymous, you might want to add a tablespoon of cocoa powder to this recipe.

YIELD: About ¾ quart

1 (13.5-ounce) can coconut milk

4 tablespoons honey

¼ teaspoon xanthan gum (optional)

3 egg yolks

1 shot of espresso

1 shot of rum

1 teaspoon vanilla extract

1 In a medium saucepan over low heat, combine coconut milk, honey, and xanthan gum (if using). Stir continuously until the mixture thickens enough to coat the back of a spoon, about 8 minutes. Set aside.

2 In a heat-safe bowl, whisk the egg yolks until they reach a fluffy consistency. Add a small ladle of the warm mixture and stir until combined. Continue adding the warm mixture, one ladle at a time, until it's completely mixed into the egg yolks. Don't add too much of the warm mixture at once or you may end up with scrambled eggs!

3 Cover the mixture and refrigerate until completely chilled (about 8 hours or up to 2 days).

4 Combine chilled mixture with espresso, rum, and vanilla extract.

5 Freeze the mixture in your ice cream maker according to the manufacturer's instructions and enjoy! If you don't plan on serving

the ice cream immediately, transfer to a freezer-proof container and freeze up to 1 week (or 2 months if you use xanthan gum and place a layer of plastic wrap on the surface of the ice cream). To serve, remove from freezer and let sit about 15 minutes, or until desired texture is reached.

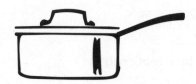

YERBA MATE ICE CREAM

Yerba mate is one of my favorite teas. As a Tim Ferriss fan, I am naturally drawn to the tea, because he credits yerba mate with the completion of *The 4-Hour Workweek*.

YIELD: About ¾ quart

1 (13.5-ounce) can coconut milk

4 tablespoons honey

¼ teaspoon xanthan gum (optional)

8 yerba mate tea bags

3 egg yolks

1   In a medium saucepan over low heat, combine coconut milk, honey, and xanthan gum (if using).

2   Add tea bags and let simmer on low heat for 30 minutes or until the ice cream reaches a mild green color, stirring occasionally. Once steeped, about 30 minutes, remove tea bags. Set aside.

3   In a heat-safe bowl, whisk the egg yolks until they reach a fluffy consistency. Add a small ladle of the warm mixture and stir until combined. Continue adding the warm mixture, one ladle at a time, until it's completely mixed into the egg yolks. Don't add too much of the warm mixture at once or you may end up with scrambled eggs!

4   Cover the mixture and refrigerate until completely chilled (about 8 hours or up to 2 days).

5   Freeze the mixture in your ice cream maker according to the manufacturer's instructions and enjoy! If you don't plan on serving the ice cream immediately, transfer to a freezer-proof container and freeze up to 1 week (or 2 months if you use xanthan gum and place a layer of plastic wrap on the surface of the ice cream). To serve, remove from freezer and let sit about 15 minutes, or until desired texture is reached.

STRAWBERRY KIWI LEMONADE ICE CREAM

Strawberry kiwi lemonade is my go-to ice cream flavor after a morning round of golf. For a truer Arnold Palmer experience, try subbing iced tea for the coconut milk.

YIELD: About 1 quart

1 (13.5-ounce) can coconut milk

4 tablespoons honey

¼ teaspoon xanthan gum (optional)

4 egg yolks

¼ cup fresh lemon juice

2 cups fresh strawberries, hulled

4 medium kiwis, peeled

1 In a medium saucepan over low heat, combine coconut milk, honey, and xanthan gum (if using). Stir continuously until the mixture thickens enough to coat the back of a spoon, about 8 minutes. Set aside.

2 In a heat-safe bowl, whisk the egg yolks until they reach a fluffy consistency. Add a small ladle of the warm mixture and stir until combined. Continue adding the warm mixture, one ladle at a time, until it's completely mixed into the egg yolks. Don't add too much of the warm mixture at once or you may end up with scrambled eggs!

3 Cover the mixture and refrigerate until completely chilled (about 8 hours or up to 2 days).

4 Blend chilled mixture with lemon juice, strawberries, and kiwis in a blender for 30 seconds or until your desired consistency is reached.

5 Freeze the mixture in your ice cream maker according to the manufacturer's instructions and enjoy! If you don't plan on serving the ice cream immediately, transfer to a freezer-proof container and

freeze up to 1 week (or 2 months if you use xanthan gum and place a layer of plastic wrap on the surface of the ice cream). To serve, remove from freezer and let sit about 15 minutes, or until desired texture is reached.

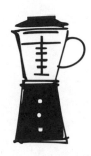

EGGNOG ICE CREAM

To make "pumpkin spice" eggnog, simply add 1 tablespoon of pumpkin pie spice in place of the other spices. If you like your eggnog to have some kick to it, stir one shot of dark rum into the mixture after it finishes cooling.

YIELD: About ¾ quart

1 (13.5-ounce) can coconut milk

4 tablespoons honey

1 tablespoon cinnamon

½ tablespoon nutmeg

¼ tablespoon cloves

¼ teaspoon xanthan gum (optional)

10 egg yolks

1 In a medium saucepan over low heat, combine coconut milk, honey, cinnamon, nutmeg, cloves, and xanthan gum (if using). Stir continuously until the mixture thickens enough to coat the back of a spoon, about 8 minutes. Set aside.

2 In a heat-safe bowl, whisk the egg yolks until they reach a fluffy consistency. Add a small ladle of the warm mixture and stir until combined. Continue adding the warm mixture, one ladle at a time, until it's completely mixed into the egg yolks. Don't add too much of the warm mixture at once or you may end up with scrambled eggs!

3 Cover the mixture and refrigerate until completely chilled (about 8 hours or up to 2 days).

4 Freeze the mixture in your ice cream maker according to the manufacturer's instructions. If you aren't serving the ice cream immediately, transfer to a freezer-proof container and freeze up to 1 week (or 2 months if you use xanthan gum and place a layer of plastic wrap on the surface of the ice cream). To serve, remove from freezer and let sit 15 minutes, or until desired texture is reached.

CHAPTER 4: SWEET INSPIRATIONS

Let's be honest. We don't make ice cream because we want to be as healthy as humanly possible. We make ice cream because every once in a while we want to indulge ourselves with one of our favorite treats! There is nothing wrong with that. Especially when our favorite treats are made up of nutrient-dense whole foods! This chapter is full of very indulgent flavors that will surely get you salivating before you even take a bite.

PUMPKIN PIE ICE CREAM

This recipe will give any pumpkin pie a run for its money and is a must-try for all pumpkin pie lovers. Though I wouldn't ever suggest replacing actual pumpkin pie on Thanksgiving (the horror!), Pumpkin Pie Ice Cream is a fun addition to the dessert selection on turkey day. Adding the homemade paleo Coconut Whipped Cream (page 161) is the perfect way to top it off.

YIELD: About ¾ quart

1 (13.5-ounce) can coconut milk

4 tablespoons honey

¼ teaspoon xanthan gum (optional)

3 egg yolks

½ cup pureed pumpkin

½ tablespoon pumpkin pie spice

1 teaspoon vanilla extract

1 In a medium saucepan over low heat, combine coconut milk, honey, and xanthan gum (if using). Stir continuously until the mixture thickens enough to coat the back of a spoon, about 8 minutes. Set aside.

2 In a heat-safe bowl, whisk the egg yolks until they reach a fluffy consistency. Add a small ladle of the warm mixture and stir until combined. Continue adding the warm mixture, one ladle at a time, until it's completely mixed into the egg yolks. Don't add too much of the warm mixture at once or you may end up with scrambled eggs!

3 Cover the mixture and refrigerate until completely chilled (about 8 hours or up to 2 days).

4 Blend chilled mixture with pureed pumpkin, pumpkin pie spice, and vanilla extract in a blender until smooth, about 30 seconds.

5 Freeze the mixture in your ice cream maker according to the manufacturer's instructions and enjoy! If you don't plan on serving

the ice cream immediately, transfer to a freezer-proof container and freeze up to 1 week (or 2 months if you use xanthan gum and place a layer of plastic wrap on the surface of the ice cream). To serve, remove from freezer and let sit about 15 minutes, or until desired texture is reached.

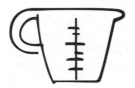

CHEESECAKE ICE CREAM

Cheesecake is one of the richest foods on the face of the planet. To be honest, this is sometimes an issue. Cheesecake tastes so good, but I can't eat more than a few bites because it fills me up so quickly. Cheesecake ice cream gives you a similar flavor without the overfilling effect. Winning! This recipe isn't strictly paleo, but it is primal and delicious.

YIELD: About 1 quart

1 (13.5-ounce) can coconut milk

4 tablespoons honey

¼ teaspoon xanthan gum (optional)

3 egg yolks

1¼ cups sour cream

1¼ cups cream cheese

1 tablespoon lemon zest

1 In a medium saucepan over low heat, combine coconut milk, honey, and xanthan gum (if using). Stir continuously until the mixture thickens enough to coat the back of a spoon, about 8 minutes. Set aside.

2 In a heat-safe bowl, whisk the egg yolks until they reach a fluffy consistency. Add a small ladle of the warm mixture and stir until combined. Continue adding the warm mixture, one ladle at a time, until it's completely mixed into the egg yolks. Don't add too much of the warm mixture at once or you may end up with scrambled eggs!

3 Cover the mixture and refrigerate until completely chilled (about 8 hours or up to 2 days).

4 Blend chilled mixture with sour cream, cream cheese, and lemon zest in a blender until smooth, about 30 seconds.

5 Freeze the mixture in your ice cream maker according to the manufacturer's instructions and enjoy! If you don't plan on serving

the ice cream immediately, transfer to a freezer-proof container and freeze up to 1 week (or 2 months if you use xanthan gum and place a layer of plastic wrap on the surface of the ice cream). To serve, remove from freezer and let sit about 15 minutes, or until desired texture is reached.

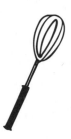

STRAWBERRY CHEESECAKE ICE CREAM

There are times when normal Cheesecake Ice Cream (page 68) is not enough. So why not add some strawberries to the mix? If you prefer, blueberries and raspberries are great in the place of the strawberries. Enjoy responsibly. The dairy in this recipe means that it also is primal rather than strict paleo.

YIELD: About 1 quart

1 (13.5-ounce) can coconut milk

4 tablespoons honey

¼ teaspoon xanthan gum (optional)

3 egg yolks

1¼ cups sour cream

1¼ cups cream cheese

1 tablespoon lemon zest

2 cups strawberry puree

1 In a medium saucepan over low heat, combine coconut milk, honey, and xanthan gum (if using). Stir continuously until the mixture thickens enough to coat the back of a spoon, about 8 minutes. Set aside.

2 In a heat-safe bowl, whisk the egg yolks until they reach a fluffy consistency. Add a small ladle of the warm mixture and stir until combined. Continue adding the warm mixture, one ladle at a time, until it's completely mixed into the egg yolks. Don't add too much of the warm mixture at once or you may end up with scrambled eggs!

3 Cover the mixture and refrigerate until completely chilled (about 8 hours or up to 2 days).

4 Blend chilled mixture with sour cream, cream cheese, and lemon zest in a blender until smooth, about 30 seconds.

5 Freeze the mixture in your ice cream maker according to the manufacturer's instructions.

6 Fold the strawberry puree into the ice cream as it begins to thicken, and enjoy. If you don't plan on serving the ice cream immediately, transfer to a freezer-proof container and freeze up to 1 week (or 2 months if you use xanthan gum and place a layer of plastic wrap on the surface of the ice cream). To serve, remove from freezer and let sit about 15 minutes, or until desired texture is reached.

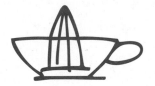

CARROT CAKE ICE CREAM

Want more vegetables in your diet? Eat more ice cream! I recommend using coconut sugar or maple syrup as the sweetener in this recipe, because they both go exceptionally well with carrots. The raisins are optional, and I personally omit them. If you like more texture in your ice cream, you can add the pecans and raisins in as the ice cream is thickening in your ice cream maker. Lastly, walnuts can be substituted for the pecans.

YIELD: About ¾ quart

¾ **cup coarsely chopped carrots**

1 **(13.5-ounce) can coconut milk**

4 **tablespoons coconut sugar**

¼ **teaspoon xanthan gum (optional)**

4 **egg yolks**

¼ **teaspoon vanilla extract**

¼ **cup cream cheese**

½ **teaspoon cinnamon**

⅛ **cup pecans**

⅛ **cup raisins**

1   Steam carrots on stovetop until soft.

2   Blend carrots with about ⅓ cup of coconut milk in a food processor until it turns into a carrot puree, about 2 minutes. Place in heat-proof container and set aside in refrigerator.

3   In a medium saucepan over low heat, combine remaining coconut milk, coconut sugar, and xanthan gum (if using). Stir continuously until the mixture thickens enough to coat the back of a spoon, about 8 minutes. Set aside.

4   In a heat-safe bowl, whisk the egg yolks until they reach a fluffy consistency. Add a small ladle of the warm mixture and stir until combined. Continue adding the warm mixture, one ladle at a time,

until it's completely mixed into the egg yolks. Don't add too much of the warm mixture at once or you may end up with scrambled eggs!

5   Cover the mixture and refrigerate until completely chilled (about 8 hours or up to 2 days).

6   Blend chilled mixture with carrot puree, vanilla extract, cream cheese, cinnamon, pecans, and raisins in a blender until the mixture becomes homogeneous, about 30 seconds.

7   Freeze the mixture in your ice cream maker according to the manufacturer's instructions and enjoy! If you don't plan on serving the ice cream immediately, transfer to a freezer-proof container and freeze up to 1 week (or 2 months if you use xanthan gum and place a layer of plastic wrap on the surface of the ice cream). To serve, remove from freezer and let sit about 15 minutes, or until desired texture is reached.

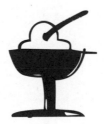

SWEET POTATO PIE ICE CREAM

Lots of folks only eat sweet potatoes in the form of crispy, salty fries. I think this insults the range of sweet potatoes, which can be used in a myriad of different dishes. Sweet potato ice cream is my little way of sticking up for the root vegetables and showing the world how versatile they are. I recommend using coconut sugar or maple syrup as the sweetener in this recipe, because they both go really well with sweet potato's flavor. Yams substitute in fine if that is what you prefer or have on hand.

YIELD: About ¾ quart

1 small sweet potato

1 (13.5-ounce) can coconut milk

4 tablespoons coconut sugar

¼ teaspoon xanthan gum (optional)

4 egg yolks

¼ cup cream cheese

1 teaspoon cinnamon

¼ teaspoon allspice

¼ teaspoon nutmeg

pinch of salt

⅛ cup walnuts

1 Cook sweet potato on a baking sheet in the oven at 350°F for 40 minutes or until soft.

2 Let cool and discard skin. Blend the sweet potato with ⅓ cup coconut milk in a food processor until it turns into a puree, about 2 minutes. Place in heat-proof container and set aside in refrigerator.

3 In a medium saucepan over low heat, combine remaining coconut milk, coconut sugar, and xanthan gum (if using). Stir continuously until the mixture thickens enough to coat the back of a spoon, about 8 minutes. Set aside.

4 In a heat-safe bowl, whisk the egg yolks until they reach a fluffy consistency. Add a small ladle of the warm mixture and stir until combined. Continue adding the warm mixture, one ladle at a time, until it's completely mixed into the egg yolks. Don't add too much of the warm mixture at once or you may end up with scrambled eggs!

5 Cover the mixture and refrigerate until completely chilled (about 8 hours or up to 2 days).

6 Blend chilled mixture with sweet potato puree, cream cheese, cinnamon, allspice, nutmeg, and salt in a blender until the mixture becomes homogeneous, about 30 seconds.

7 Freeze the mixture in your ice cream maker according to the manufacturer's instructions.

8 Fold walnuts into the ice cream as it begins to thicken in your ice cream machine and enjoy! If you don't plan on serving the ice cream immediately, transfer to a freezer-proof container and freeze up to 1 week (or 2 months if you use xanthan gum and place a layer of plastic wrap on the surface of the ice cream). To serve, remove from freezer and let sit about 15 minutes, or until desired texture is reached.

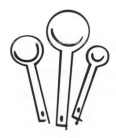

MIXED BERRY PIE ICE CREAM

Growing up in Seattle, I had access to wild salmonberries every summer and am very fond of the fruit. If they are too difficult to obtain, you can simply omit them and use more blackberries and raspberries or substitute strawberries or blueberries. The flavor will certainly change, but your ice cream will taste just as good! There isn't a bad berry combination out there, so try as many combinations and varieties as you can get your hands on.

YIELD: About 1 quart

½ **tablespoon butter**

⅔ **cup raspberries**

⅔ **cup blackberries**

⅔ **cup salmonberries**

½ **tablespoon freshly squeezed lemon juice**

½ **tablespoon coconut flour**

½ **tablespoon almond flour**

1 **(13.5-ounce) can coconut milk**

4 **tablespoons honey**

¼ **teaspoon xanthan gum (optional)**

4 **egg yolks**

1 Melt the butter in a large skillet over low heat.

2 Add raspberries, blackberries, salmonberries, lemon juice, coconut flour, and almond flour and sauté for two minutes or until the berries are very soft. Place in heat-proof container and set aside in refrigerator.

3 In a medium saucepan over low heat, combine coconut milk, honey, and xanthan gum (if using). Stir continuously until the mixture thickens enough to coat the back of a spoon, about 8 minutes. Set aside.

4   In a heat-safe bowl, whisk the egg yolks until they reach a fluffy consistency. Add a small ladle of the warm mixture and stir until combined. Continue adding the warm mixture, one ladle at a time, until it's completely mixed into the egg yolks. Don't add too much of the warm mixture at once or you may end up with scrambled eggs!

5   Cover the mixture and refrigerate until completely chilled (about 8 hours or up to 2 days).

6   Blend chilled mixture with the berries until smooth.

7   Freeze the mixture in your ice cream maker according to the manufacturer's instructions and enjoy! If you don't plan on serving the ice cream immediately, transfer to a freezer-proof container and freeze up to 1 week (or 2 months if you use xanthan gum and place a layer of plastic wrap on the surface of the ice cream). To serve, remove from freezer and let sit about 15 minutes, or until desired texture is reached.

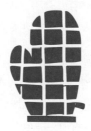

CANDY BAR ICE CREAM

Growing up, I loved candy bars. These days, their flavor is way too overpowering for my mature, twenty-one-year-old taste buds. Candy Bar Ice Cream is a way for me to get that nutty, chocolaty flavor without feeling like I just ate a box of sugar cubes.

YIELD: About ¾ quart

1 ⅔ cups almond milk

4 tablespoons honey

¼ teaspoon xanthan gum (optional)

4 egg yolks

¼ cup almond butter

2 tablespoons cocoa powder

2 teaspoons vanilla extract

¼ cup toasted almonds

⅛ cup Caramel (page 155)

1   In a medium saucepan over low heat, combine almond milk, honey, and xanthan gum (if using). Stir continuously until the mixture thickens enough to coat the back of a spoon, about 8 minutes. Set aside.

2   In a heat-safe bowl, whisk the egg yolks until they reach a fluffy consistency. Add a small ladle of the warm mixture and stir until combined. Continue adding the warm mixture, one ladle at a time, until it's completely mixed into the egg yolks. Don't add too much of the warm mixture at once or you may end up with scrambled eggs!

3   Cover the mixture and refrigerate until completely chilled (about 8 hours or up to 2 days).

4   Blend chilled mixture with almond butter, cocoa powder, and vanilla extract until a homogeneous texture is achieved, about 30 seconds.

4 Freeze the mixture in your ice cream maker according to the manufacturer's instructions.

5 Midway through the ice cream's thickening process, sprinkle the toasted almonds and Caramel in and enjoy! If you don't plan on serving the ice cream immediately, transfer to a freezer-proof container and freeze up to 1 week (or 2 months if you use xanthan gum and place a layer of plastic wrap on the surface of the ice cream). To serve, remove from freezer and let sit about 15 minutes, or until desired texture is reached.

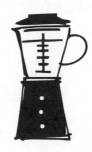

DOUBLE CHOCOLATE CANDY BAR ICE CREAM

What is better than a candy bar with one type of chocolate? Yeah, that's right, a candy bar with two types of chocolate. If you don't want to expend the money and time to obtain cacao nibs, using a crushed, unsweetened baking chocolate bar works too.

YIELD: About ¾ quart

1 ⅔ cups almond milk

4 tablespoons honey

¼ teaspoon xanthan gum (optional)

4 egg yolks

¼ cup almond butter

2 teaspoons vanilla extract

¼ cup toasted almonds

⅛ cup crushed chocolate bar pieces

⅛ cup cacao nibs

⅛ cup Caramel (page 155)

1 In a medium saucepan over low heat, combine almond milk, honey, and xanthan gum (if using). Stir continuously until the mixture thickens enough to coat the back of a spoon, about 8 minutes. Set aside.

2 In a heat-safe bowl, whisk the egg yolks until they reach a fluffy consistency. Add a small ladle of the warm mixture and stir until combined. Continue adding the warm mixture, one ladle at a time, until it's completely mixed into the egg yolks. Don't add too much of the warm mixture at once or you may end up with scrambled eggs!

3 Cover the mixture and refrigerate until completely chilled (about 8 hours or up to 2 days).

4 Blend chilled mixture with almond butter and vanilla extract in a blender, until a homogeneous texture is achieved, about 30 seconds.

4 Freeze the mixture in your ice cream maker according to the manufacturer's instructions.

5 Midway through the ice cream's thickening process, sprinkle the toasted almonds, crushed chocolate bar pieces, cacao nibs, and Caramel in and enjoy! If you don't plan on serving the ice cream immediately, transfer to a freezer-proof container and freeze up to 1 week (or 2 months if you use xanthan gum and place a layer of plastic wrap on the surface of the ice cream). To serve, remove from freezer and let sit about 15 minutes, or until desired texture is reached.

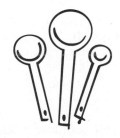

APPLE PIE ICE CREAM

No other recipe in this book inspires as much patriotism as Apple Pie Ice Cream. You can try using maple syrup or honey, but coconut sugar is definitely my recommendation. Listening to Don McLean while whipping this one up is optional but encouraged.

YIELD: About 1 quart

2 tablespoons butter

1 tablespoon cinnamon

½ teaspoon nutmeg

½ teaspoon cloves

½ tablespoon coconut flour

½ tablespoon almond flour

2 apples, peeled and thinly sliced

1 (13.5-ounce) can coconut milk

4 tablespoons coconut sugar

¼ teaspoon xanthan gum (optional)

2 teaspoons vanilla extract

4 egg yolks

1 Melt butter in a large skillet over low heat. Set aside.

2 Add cinnamon, nutmeg, cloves, coconut flour, almond flour, and apples and sauté for five minutes or until soft. Place in heat-proof container and set aside in refrigerator.

3 In a medium saucepan over low heat, combine coconut milk, coconut sugar, xanthan gum (if using), and vanilla extract. Stir continuously until the mixture thickens enough to coat the back of a spoon, about 8 minutes. Set aside.

4 In a heat-safe bowl, whisk the egg yolks until they reach a fluffy consistency. Add a small ladle of the warm mixture and stir until combined. Continue adding the warm mixture, one ladle at a time,

until it's completely mixed into the egg yolks. Don't add too much of the warm mixture at once or you may end up with scrambled eggs!

5   Cover the mixture and refrigerate until completely chilled (about 8 hours or up to 2 days).

6   Blend the chilled mixture with the apples until smooth, about 30 seconds.

7   Freeze the mixture in your ice cream maker according to the manufacturer's instructions and enjoy! If you don't plan on serving the ice cream immediately, transfer to a freezer-proof container and freeze up to 1 week (or 2 months if you use xanthan gum and place a layer of plastic wrap on the surface of the ice cream). To serve, remove from freezer and let sit about 15 minutes, or until desired texture is reached.

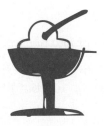

STRAWBERRY BROWNIE SUNDAE ICE CREAM

Topping this flavor off with Coconut Whipped Cream (page 161) and Strawberry Sauce (page 153) makes this recipe even more luxurious. Folks who like crunch might also want to include some toasted nuts in this one as well.

YIELD: About 1 quart

1 (13.5-ounce) can coconut milk

3 tablespoons honey

¼ teaspoon xanthan gum (optional)

2 teaspoons vanilla extract

3 egg yolks

1 cup Brownie crumbles (page 154)

¼ cup Chocolate Sauce (page 149)

1 cup fresh strawberries, sliced

1 In a medium saucepan over low heat, combine coconut milk, honey, xanthan gum (if using), and vanilla extract. Stir continuously until the mixture thickens enough to coat the back of a spoon, about 8 minutes. Set aside.

2 In a heat-safe bowl, whisk the egg yolks until they reach a fluffy consistency. Add a small ladle of the warm mixture and stir until combined. Continue adding the warm mixture, one ladle at a time, until it's completely mixed into the egg yolks. Don't add too much of the warm mixture at once or you may end up with scrambled eggs!

3 Cover the mixture and refrigerate until completely chilled (about 8 hours or up to 2 days).

4 Make a batch of Brownies, and crumble them into small pieces with a fork.

5   Freeze the ice cream mixture in your ice cream maker according to the manufacturer's instructions.

6   When ice cream is nearly done thickening, pour the Chocolate Sauce into the ice cream machine along with the strawberry slices and Brownie crumbles and enjoy! If you don't plan on serving the ice cream immediately, transfer to a freezer-proof container and freeze up to 1 week (or 2 months if you use xanthan gum and place a layer of plastic wrap on the surface of the ice cream). To serve, remove from freezer and let sit about 15 minutes, or until desired texture is reached.

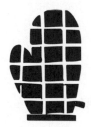

BANANA CREAM PIE ICE CREAM

You can spruce up the appearance and taste of this recipe by putting a dash of cocoa powder on top of your scoop. I have to admit, I've never actually eaten banana cream pie. If it tastes anything like this ice cream, though, then I am very much in support of it.

YIELD: About 1¼ quarts

1 tablespoon butter

2 teaspoons vanilla extract

4 ripe, mashed bananas

⅛ teaspoon lemon juice

¼ teaspoon nutmeg

½ tablespoon coconut flour

½ tablespoon almond flour

1 (13.5-ounce) can coconut milk

2 tablespoons honey

¼ teaspoon xanthan gum (optional)

3 egg yolks

1 Melt butter in a large skillet over low heat.

2 Add vanilla extract, mashed bananas, lemon juice, nutmeg, coconut flour, and almond flour and then sauté the banana mixture for one minute. Place in heat-proof container and set aside in refrigerator.

3 In a medium saucepan over low heat, combine coconut milk, honey, and xanthan gum (if using). Stir continuously until the mixture thickens enough to coat the back of a spoon, about 8 minutes. Set aside.

4 In a heat-safe bowl, whisk the egg yolks until they reach a fluffy consistency. Add a small ladle of the warm mixture and stir until

combined. Continue adding the warm mixture, one ladle at a time, until it's completely mixed into the egg yolks. Don't add too much of the warm mixture at once or you may end up with scrambled eggs!

5 Cover the mixture and refrigerate until completely chilled (about 8 hours or up to 2 days).

6 Blend chilled mixture with the banana mixture until smooth, about 30 seconds.

7 Freeze the mixture in your ice cream maker according to the manufacturer's instructions and enjoy! If you don't plan on serving the ice cream immediately, transfer to a freezer-proof container and freeze up to 1 week (or 2 months if you use xanthan gum and place a layer of plastic wrap on the surface of the ice cream). To serve, remove from freezer and let sit about 15 minutes, or until desired texture is reached.

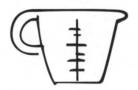

CHAPTER 5: ADVENTUROUS FLAVORS

Just because ice cream is a common treat doesn't mean it can't be made with uncommon ingredients! After you scratch your itch for more traditional ice cream flavors, give these unusual flavors a spin.

SALTED CARAMEL ICE CREAM

If you like caramel but have refrained from eating it in an attempt to stay strict paleo, you are missing out, my friend. Every time I make homemade caramel, it ends up disappearing more quickly than I anticipate. Don't say I didn't warn you.

YIELD: About ¾ quart

1 (13.5-ounce) can coconut milk

3 tablespoons honey

¼ teaspoon xanthan gum (optional)

3 egg yolks

½ teaspoon salt

¼ cup Caramel (page 155)

1 In a medium saucepan over low heat, combine coconut milk, honey, and xanthan gum (if using). Stir continuously until the mixture thickens enough to coat the back of a spoon, about 8 minutes. Set aside.

2 In a heat-safe bowl, whisk the egg yolks until they reach a fluffy consistency. Add a small ladle of the warm mixture and stir until combined. Continue adding the warm mixture, one ladle at a time, until it's completely mixed into the egg yolks. Don't add too much of the warm mixture at once or you may end up with scrambled eggs!

3 Cover the mixture and refrigerate until completely chilled (about 8 hours or up to 2 days).

4 Freeze the mixture in your ice cream maker according to the manufacturer's instructions.

5 Midway through the ice cream's thickening process, mix salt into the Caramel and then drizzle the mixture into the ice cream. If you don't plan on serving the ice cream immediately, transfer to a

freezer-proof container and freeze up to 1 week (or 2 months if you use xanthan gum and place a layer of plastic wrap on the surface of the ice cream). To serve, remove from freezer and let sit about 15 minutes, or until desired texture is reached.

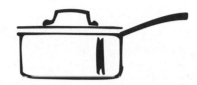

CAYENNE CHOCOLATE ICE CREAM

If you like spicy food, this is definitely the flavor for you. Just be careful because a little bit of cayenne goes a long way.

YIELD: About ¾ quart

1 (13.5-ounce) can coconut milk

4 tablespoons honey

¼ teaspoon xanthan gum (optional)

2 tablespoons cocoa powder

¼ teaspoon cayenne pepper

3 egg yolks

1 In a medium saucepan over low heat, combine coconut milk, honey, xanthan gum (if using), cocoa powder, and cayenne pepper. Stir continuously until the mixture thickens enough to coat the back of a spoon, about 8 minutes. Set aside.

2 In a heat-safe bowl, whisk the egg yolks until they reach a fluffy consistency. Add a small ladle of the warm mixture and stir until combined. Continue adding the warm mixture, one ladle at a time, until it's completely mixed into the egg yolks. Don't add too much of the warm mixture at once or you may end up with scrambled eggs!

3 Cover the mixture and refrigerate until completely chilled (about 8 hours or up to 2 days).

4 Freeze the mixture in your ice cream maker according to the manufacturer's instructions. If you aren't serving the ice cream immediately, transfer to a freezer-proof container and freeze up to 1 week (or 2 months if you use xanthan gum and place a layer of plastic wrap on the surface of the ice cream). To serve, remove from freezer and let sit 15 minutes, or until desired texture is reached.

OREGANO ICE CREAM

This ice cream will work with a number of herbs and spices, including lavender, saffron, and cardamom. You can even use cannabis, if it is legal in your state.

YIELD: About ¾ quart

1 (13.5-ounce) can coconut milk

4 tablespoons honey

¼ teaspoon xanthan gum (optional)

¼ cup fresh oregano leaves

3 egg yolks

1 In a medium saucepan over low heat, combine coconut milk, honey, and xanthan gum (if using).

2 Add the oregano and let simmer on low heat for about an hour, stirring occasionally. Once steeped, strain the warm mixture through a fine-mesh strainer in order to remove the leaves. Set aside.

3 In a heat-safe bowl, whisk the egg yolks until they reach a fluffy consistency. Add a small ladle of the warm mixture and stir until combined. Continue adding the warm mixture, one ladle at a time, until it's completely mixed into the egg yolks. Don't add too much of the warm mixture at once or you may end up with scrambled eggs!

4 Cover the mixture and refrigerate until completely chilled (about 8 hours or up to 2 days).

5 Freeze the mixture in your ice cream maker according to the manufacturer's instructions and enjoy! If you don't plan on serving the ice cream immediately, transfer to a freezer-proof container and freeze up to 1 week (or 2 months if you use xanthan gum and place a layer of plastic wrap on the surface of the ice cream). To serve, remove from freezer and let sit about 15 minutes, or until desired texture is reached.

GOAT CHEESE ICE CREAM

Goat cheese ice cream is woefully underappreciated. This primal flavor is simultaneously exotic and classy while still being extremely easy to eat.

YIELD: About ¾ quart

1 (13.5-ounce) can coconut milk

4 tablespoons honey

¼ teaspoon xanthan gum (optional)

3 egg yolks

¼ cup goat cheese

1 In a medium saucepan over low heat, combine coconut milk, honey, and xanthan gum (if using). Stir continuously until the mixture thickens enough to coat the back of a spoon, about 8 minutes. Set aside.

2 In a heat-safe bowl, whisk the egg yolks until they reach a fluffy consistency. Add a small ladle of the warm mixture and stir until combined. Continue adding the warm mixture, one ladle at a time, until it's completely mixed into the egg yolks. Don't add too much of the warm mixture at once or you may end up with scrambled eggs!

3 Cover the mixture and refrigerate until completely chilled (about 8 hours or up to 2 days).

4 Blend mixture with the goat cheese in blender until smooth, about 30 seconds.

5 Freeze the mixture in your ice cream maker according to the manufacturer's instructions. If you don't serve the ice cream immediately, transfer to a freezer-proof container and freeze up to 1 week (or 2 months if you use xanthan gum and place a layer of plastic wrap on the surface of the ice cream). To serve, remove from freezer and let sit 15 minutes, or until desired texture is reached.

OLIVE OIL ICE CREAM

Though olive oil doesn't sound like it would work very well as an ice cream flavor, it is very tasty, especially after an Italian dinner.

YIELD: About ¾ quart

1 (13.5-ounce) can coconut milk

4 tablespoons honey

¼ teaspoon xanthan gum (optional)

3 egg yolks

½ cup olive oil

¾ teaspoon salt

1 In a medium saucepan over low heat, combine coconut milk, honey, and xanthan gum (if using). Stir continuously until the mixture thickens enough to coat the back of a spoon, about 8 minutes. Set aside.

2 In a heat-safe bowl, whisk the egg yolks until they reach a fluffy consistency. Add a small ladle of the warm mixture and stir until combined. Continue adding the warm mixture, one ladle at a time, until it's completely mixed into the egg yolks. Don't add too much of the warm mixture at once or you may end up with scrambled eggs!

3 Stir in olive oil and salt.

4 Cover the mixture and refrigerate until completely chilled (about 8 hours or up to 2 days).

5 Freeze the mixture in your ice cream maker according to the manufacturer's instructions and enjoy! If you don't plan on serving the ice cream immediately, transfer to a freezer-proof container and freeze up to 1 week (or 2 months if you use xanthan gum and place a layer of plastic wrap on the surface of the ice cream). To serve, remove from freezer and let sit 15 minutes, or until desired texture is reached.

CUCUMBER MINT ICE CREAM

This flavor is for the folks who like green smoothies. It is different, yet refreshing and decidedly tasty. A fantastic summer recipe!

YIELD: About ¾ quart

1 (13.5-ounce) can coconut milk

4 tablespoons honey

¼ teaspoon xanthan gum (optional)

4 egg yolks

1 teaspoon peppermint extract

1 large, chopped cucumber

1　In a medium saucepan over low heat, combine coconut milk, honey, and xanthan gum (if using). Stir continuously until the mixture thickens enough to coat the back of a spoon, about 8 minutes. Set aside.

2　In a heat-safe bowl, whisk the egg yolks until they reach a fluffy consistency. Add a small ladle of the warm mixture and stir until combined. Continue adding the warm mixture, one ladle at a time, until it's completely mixed into the egg yolks. Don't add too much of the warm mixture at once or you may end up with scrambled eggs!

3　Cover the mixture and refrigerate until completely chilled (about 8 hours or up to 2 days).

4　Blend chilled mixture with peppermint extract and cucumber in a blender for 30 seconds or until a smooth texture is reached.

5　Freeze the mixture in your ice cream maker according to the manufacturer's instructions and enjoy! If you don't plan on serving the ice cream immediately, transfer to a freezer-proof container and freeze up to 1 week (or 2 months if you use xanthan gum and place a layer of plastic wrap on the surface of the ice cream). To serve, remove from freezer and let sit about 15 minutes, or until desired texture is reached.

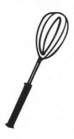

BLACK LICORICE ICE CREAM

People are either die-hard fans or completely opposed to the taste of black licorice. I think adding some vanilla to the anise makes it more accessible for the general population without detracting from its core flavor. Hopefully, this Black Licorice Ice Cream falls into your "love it" category.

YIELD: About ¾ quart

1 (13.5-ounce) can coconut milk

4 tablespoons honey

¼ teaspoon xanthan gum (optional)

1 teaspoon vanilla extract

¼ cup anise or star anise

3 egg yolks

1   In a medium saucepan over low heat, combine coconut milk, honey, xanthan gum (if using), and vanilla extract.

2   Add anise and let simmer on low heat for 45 minutes, stirring occasionally. Once steeped, strain the warm mixture through a fine-mesh strainer in order to remove the anise.

3   In a heat-safe bowl, whisk the egg yolks until they reach a fluffy consistency. Add a small ladle of the warm mixture and stir until combined. Continue adding the warm mixture, one ladle at a time, until it's completely mixed into the egg yolks. Don't add too much of the warm mixture at once or you may end up with scrambled eggs!

4   Cover the mixture and refrigerate until completely chilled (about 8 hours or up to 2 days).

5   Freeze the mixture in your ice cream maker according to the manufacturer's instructions and enjoy! If you don't plan on serving the ice cream immediately, transfer to a freezer-proof container and

freeze up to 1 week (or 2 months if you use xanthan gum and place a layer of plastic wrap on the surface of the ice cream). To serve, remove from freezer and let sit about 15 minutes, or until desired texture is reached.

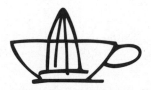

CHOCOLATE STOUT ICE CREAM

If you like chocolate stout, or really any beer for that matter, try this recipe when in an adventurous mood. No, stout beer isn't strictly a paleo-approved choice, but beer has been consumed for thousands of years. If you are not gluten-insensitive, I don't think a little Chocolate Stout Ice Cream will pose a threat to your healthy lifestyle.

YIELD: About ¾ quart

1 (13.5-ounce) can coconut milk

4 tablespoons honey

¼ teaspoon xanthan gum (optional)

4 egg yolks

1½ tablespoons cocoa powder

1 teaspoon vanilla extract

½ cup stout beer

1 In a medium saucepan over low heat, combine coconut milk, honey, and xanthan gum (if using). Stir continuously until the mixture thickens enough to coat the back of a spoon, about 8 minutes. Set aside.

2 In a heat-safe bowl, whisk the egg yolks until they reach a fluffy consistency. Add a small ladle of the warm mixture and stir until combined. Continue adding the warm mixture, one ladle at a time, until it's completely mixed into the egg yolks. Don't add too much of the warm mixture at once or you may end up with scrambled eggs!

3 Cover the mixture and refrigerate until completely chilled (about 8 hours or up to 2 days).

4 Blend chilled mixture with cocoa powder, vanilla extract, and stout in a blender until completely combined, about 20 seconds.

5 Freeze the mixture in your ice cream maker according to the manufacturer's instructions and enjoy! If you don't plan on serving the ice cream immediately, transfer to a freezer-proof container and freeze up to 1 week (or 2 months if you use xanthan gum and place a layer of plastic wrap on the surface of the ice cream). To serve, remove from freezer and let sit about 15 minutes, or until desired texture is reached.

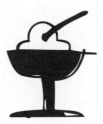

BLACK PEPPERCORN ICE CREAM

Growing up, I couldn't stand even a small amount of pepper sprinkled on my food, much to the dismay of my dad. These days, I pour the stuff on until there is a nice, black layer atop my dish. Including a pepper ice cream flavor in this book should be the final step to get me back in the pepper god's good graces. Try this recipe if you are in the mood for an exotic indulgence.

YIELD: About ¾ quart

1 (13.5-ounce) can coconut milk

4 tablespoons honey

pinch of salt

¼ teaspoon xanthan gum (optional)

1 tablespoon cracked black peppercorns

3 egg yolks

1 In a medium saucepan over low heat, combine coconut milk, honey, salt, and xanthan gum (if using).

2 Add cracked black peppercorns and let simmer on low heat for half an hour, stirring occasionally. Once steeped, strain the warm mixture through a fine-mesh strainer in order to remove the cracked peppercorns.

3 In a heat-safe bowl, whisk the egg yolks until they reach a fluffy consistency. Add a small ladle of the warm mixture and stir until combined. Continue adding the warm mixture, one ladle at a time, until it's completely mixed into the egg yolks. Don't add too much of the warm mixture at once or you may end up with scrambled eggs!

4 Cover the mixture and refrigerate until completely chilled (about 8 hours or up to 2 days).

5 Freeze the mixture in your ice cream maker according to the manufacturer's instructions and enjoy! If you don't plan on serving the ice cream immediately, transfer to a freezer-proof container and freeze up to 1 week (or 2 months if you use xanthan gum and place a layer of plastic wrap on the surface of the ice cream). To serve, remove from freezer and let sit about 15 minutes, or until desired texture is reached.

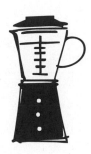

MAPLE CHOCOLATE BACON ICE CREAM

Maple syrup? Good! Chocolate? Good! Bacon? Good! This flavor should definitely appeal to the sweet and salty crowd that likes maple syrup on their sausages in the morning.

YIELD: About ¾ quart

1 (13.5-ounce) can coconut milk

4 tablespoons maple syrup

¼ teaspoon xanthan gum (optional)

3 egg yolks

1 batch Chocolate Pieces (page 148)

3 strips of crispy bacon, dried well with paper towels and cut into ½-inch pieces

1 In a medium saucepan over low heat, combine coconut milk, maple syrup, and xanthan gum (if using). Stir continuously until the mixture thickens enough to coat the back of a spoon, about 8 minutes. Set aside.

2 In a heat-safe bowl, whisk the egg yolks until they reach a fluffy consistency. Add a small ladle of the warm mixture and stir until combined. Continue adding the warm mixture, one ladle at a time, until it's completely mixed into the egg yolks. Don't add too much of the warm mixture at once or you may end up with scrambled eggs!

3 Cover the mixture and refrigerate until completely chilled (about 8 hours or up to 2 days).

4 Follow steps 1 through 3 in the Chocolate Pieces recipe (page 148). Before the chocolate cools, stir in the crispy bacon pieces. Then pour the chocolate-covered bacon pieces onto a baking sheet lined with waxed paper and let stand until completely cooled.

5 Freeze the ice cream mixture in your ice cream maker according to the manufacturer's instructions.

6 Sprinkle in the chocolate-covered bacon pieces midway through the ice cream's thickening process. If you don't plan on serving the ice cream immediately, transfer to a freezer-proof container and freeze up to 1 week (or 2 months if you use xanthan gum and place a layer of plastic wrap on the surface of the ice cream). To serve, remove from freezer and let sit about 15 minutes, or until desired texture is reached.

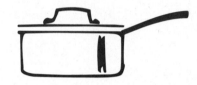

CHOCOLATE POMEGRANATE ICE CREAM

Pomegranate juice, vodka, and chocolate are an unlikely trio. With an open mind, I think you'll find that the combination works quite well, however. If you like the crunch that pomegranate seeds provide, you can toss them in the mix, too.

YIELD: About ¾ quart

1 (13.5-ounce) can coconut milk

4 tablespoons honey

¼ teaspoon xanthan gum (optional)

5 egg yolks

2 cups pomegranate juice

1 teaspoon vodka

¼ cup Chocolate Sauce (page 149)

1   In a medium saucepan over low heat, combine coconut milk, honey, and xanthan gum (if using). Stir continuously until the mixture thickens enough to coat the back of a spoon, about 8 minutes. Set aside.

2   In a heat-safe bowl, whisk the egg yolks until they reach a fluffy consistency. Add a small ladle of the warm mixture and stir until combined. Continue adding the warm mixture, one ladle at a time, until it's completely mixed into the egg yolks. Don't add too much of the warm mixture at once or you may end up with scrambled eggs!

3   Cover the mixture and refrigerate until completely chilled (about 8 hours or up to 2 days).

4   Blend chilled mixture, pomegranate juice, and vodka in a blender until smooth, about 15 seconds.

5 Freeze the mixture in your ice cream maker according to the manufacturer's instructions.

6 Midway through the ice cream's thickening process, pour the Chocolate Sauce into the mix and enjoy! If you don't plan on serving the ice cream immediately, transfer to a freezer-proof container and freeze up to 1 week (or 2 months if you use xanthan gum and place a layer of plastic wrap on the surface of the ice cream). To serve, remove from freezer and let sit about 15 minutes, or until desired texture is reached.

SUNFLOWER SEED BUTTER AND JELLY ICE CREAM

If you want to use an additive-free peanut butter in this recipe, you can. I promise I won't tell the Paleo Police! If you have a peanut allergy or just don't do well with the stuff but want a similar flavor, I think sunflower seed butter is the most apt replacement. Feel free to experiment with other nut butters, too, if you want. If you don't mind a bit of added sugar, substituting actual jam makes this flavor taste even more like your favorite childhood sandwich. Raspberries will work just as well as strawberries, so if those are your preferred berry, use 'em!

YIELD: About 1 quart

1 ⅔ cups almond milk

3 tablespoons honey

¼ teaspoon xanthan gum (optional)

4 egg yolks

2 cups fresh strawberries, hulled

½ cup sunflower seed butter

1 In a medium saucepan over low heat, combine almond milk, honey, and xanthan gum (if using). Stir continuously until the mixture thickens enough to coat the back of a spoon, about 8 minutes. Set aside.

2 In a heat-safe bowl, whisk the egg yolks until they reach a fluffy consistency. Add a small ladle of the warm mixture and stir until combined. Continue adding the warm mixture, one ladle at a time, until it's completely mixed into the egg yolks. Don't add too much of the warm mixture at once or you may end up with scrambled eggs!

3 Cover the mixture and refrigerate until completely chilled (about 8 hours or up to 2 days).

4 Blend chilled mixture with strawberries until smooth, about 30 seconds.

5 Freeze the mixture in your ice cream maker according to the manufacturer's instructions.

6 Midway through the ice cream's thickening process, drizzle in sunflower seed butter and enjoy! If you don't plan on serving the ice cream immediately, transfer to a freezer-proof container and freeze up to 1 week (or 2 months if you use xanthan gum and place a layer of plastic wrap on the surface of the ice cream). To serve, remove from freezer and let sit about 15 minutes, or until desired texture is reached.

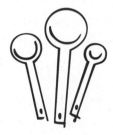

PISTACHIO ICE CREAM

Pistachio gelato is a common flavor in Italy, and for good reason. It tastes fantastic!

YIELD: About ¾ quart

1 ⅔ cups almond milk

4 tablespoons honey

¼ teaspoon xanthan gum (optional)

¼ teaspoon almond extract

¼ teaspoon vanilla extract

4 egg yolks

½ cup shelled, finely ground pistachios

1 In a medium saucepan over low heat, combine almond milk, honey, xanthan gum (if using), almond extract, and vanilla extract. Stir continuously until the mixture thickens enough to coat the back of a spoon, about 8 minutes. Set aside.

2 In a heat-safe bowl, whisk the egg yolks until they reach a fluffy consistency. Add a small ladle of the warm mixture and stir until combined. Continue adding the warm mixture, one ladle at a time, until it's completely mixed into the egg yolks. Don't add too much of the warm mixture at once or you may end up with scrambled eggs!

3 Cover the mixture and refrigerate until completely chilled (about 8 hours or up to 2 days).

4 Mix chilled mixture with pistachios in a blender for 30 seconds.

5 Freeze the mixture in your ice cream maker according to the manufacturer's instructions. If you don't serve the ice cream immediately, transfer to a freezer-proof container and freeze up to 1 week (or 2 months if you use xanthan gum and place a layer of plastic wrap on the surface of the ice cream). To serve, remove from freezer and let sit 15 minutes, or until desired texture is reached.

CHAPTER 6: SORBETS

On a warm day, there is nothing better than a refreshing scoop of homemade sorbet. Sorbet even works well in the winter, when you are craving warm weather and warm-weather treats. Come to think of it, sorbet makes for a delicious dessert all year round!

LEMON SORBET

Lemon Sorbet provides the ultimate sweet and sour experience. Therefore, this recipe is devoted to all of the recovering Sour Patch Kids addicts out there. With this recipe and all of the other recipes that call for orange or lemon zest, ideally, organic fruits will be used. Many nonorganic lemons and oranges are sprayed with things you don't want to put in your body, so if you do end up using nonorganic citrus fruits, make sure to wash them thoroughly.

YIELD: About ¾ quart

1 ⅔ cups water

4 tablespoons honey

¼ teaspoon xanthan gum (optional)

½ cup fresh lemon juice

1 tablespoon freshly grated lemon zest

1   In a blender, blend all ingredients together until mixture is uniform, about 30 seconds.

2   Cover the mixture and refrigerate until completely chilled (about 8 hours or up to 2 days).

3   Freeze the mixture in your ice cream maker according to the manufacturer's instructions and enjoy! If you don't plan on serving the sorbet immediately, transfer to a freezer-proof container and freeze up to 1 week (or 2 months if you use xanthan gum and place a layer of plastic wrap on the surface of the ice cream). To serve, remove from freezer and let sit about 15 minutes, or until desired texture is reached.

WATERMELON SORBET

Everyone loves eating watermelon in the summer but not too many people make their own watermelon sorbet. If that is you, be sure to try this recipe out on a warm, summer night. You can omit the lemon juice for a truer watermelon flavor or keep it for a bit more complexity. You can also add a shot or two of vodka to add even more layers of flavor to the recipe.

YIELD: About 1 quart

1 ⅔ cups water

2 tablespoons honey

¼ teaspoon xanthan gum (optional)

1 tablespoon fresh lemon juice

1½ cups fresh seedless watermelon

1 In a blender, blend all ingredients together until mixture is uniform, about 30 seconds.

2 Cover the mixture and refrigerate until completely chilled (about 8 hours or up to 2 days).

3 Freeze the mixture in your ice cream maker according to the manufacturer's instructions and enjoy! If you don't plan on serving the sorbet immediately, transfer to a freezer-proof container and freeze up to 1 week (or 2 months if you use xanthan gum and place a layer of plastic wrap on the surface of the ice cream). To serve, remove from freezer and let sit about 15 minutes, or until desired texture is reached.

BLACKBERRY SORBET

Wild blackberry picking is quite good in my hometown of Seattle. I've never been able to make ice cream with handpicked berries, though, because they always seem to disappear before I get home. Also, if you happen to be one of the lucky people with access to huckleberries, they taste exceedingly delicious in ice cream.

YIELD: About 1 quart

1 ⅔ cups water

3 tablespoons honey

¼ teaspoon xanthan gum (optional)

2 cups ripe blackberries

1   In a blender, blend all ingredients together until mixture is uniform, about 30 seconds.

2   Cover the mixture and refrigerate until completely chilled (about 8 hours or up to 2 days).

3   Freeze the mixture in your ice cream maker according to the manufacturer's instructions and enjoy! If you don't plan on serving the sorbet immediately, transfer to a freezer-proof container and freeze up to 1 week (or 2 months if you use xanthan gum and place a layer of plastic wrap on the surface of the ice cream). To serve, remove from freezer and let sit about 15 minutes, or until desired texture is reached.

MANGO SORBET

A small splash of brandy can bring out the flavor of mangoes and is a good optional addition to mango ice cream. Mangoes are one of those fruits where being fresh really makes a difference in flavor and sweetness. If only the mouth-watering mangoes I ate in the Canary Islands grew in Seattle.

YIELD: About 1 quart

1 ⅔ cups water

3 tablespoons honey

¼ teaspoon xanthan gum (optional)

1 large ripe mango, cored and peeled

1 In a blender, blend all ingredients together until mixture is uniform, about 30 seconds.

2 Cover the mixture and refrigerate until completely chilled (about 8 hours or up to 2 days).

3 Freeze the mixture in your ice cream maker according to the manufacturer's instructions and enjoy! If you don't plan on serving the sorbet immediately, transfer to a freezer-proof container and freeze up to 1 week (2 months if you use xanthan gum and place a layer of plastic wrap on the surface of the ice cream). To serve, remove from freezer and let sit about 15 minutes, or until desired texture is reached.

GINGER SORBET

Though a lot of people think of ginger as a complementary flavor, it can be the main act as well. This ice cream flavor is a perfect example of ginger's ability to play lead and will be a favorite for fans of the popular chewy ginger candies.

YIELD: About ¾ quart

1 ⅔ cups water

3 tablespoons honey

¼ teaspoon xanthan gum (optional)

1 large ginger root, peeled and thinly sliced

1 In a medium saucepan over low heat, combine water, honey, and xanthan gum (if using).

2 Add ginger and let simmer on low until desired strength of flavor is reached, about 15 minutes. Once steeped, strain with a fine-mesh strainer to remove ginger slices.

3 Cover the mixture and refrigerate until completely chilled (about 8 hours or up to 2 days).

4 Freeze the mixture in your ice cream maker according to the manufacturer's instructions and enjoy! If you don't plan on serving the sorbet immediately, transfer to a freezer-proof container and freeze up to 1 week (or 2 months if you use xanthan gum and place a layer of plastic wrap on the surface of the ice cream). To serve, remove from freezer and let sit about 15 minutes, or until desired texture is reached.

ALMOND CHIP SORBET

I think the flavor of almond is tragically underrated. Something needs to put a stop to this disrespect, and I think Almond Chip Sorbet might be up to the job.

YIELD: About 1 quart

1 ⅔ cups almond milk

3 tablespoons honey

¼ teaspoon xanthan gum (optional)

1 teaspoon almond extract

1 teaspoon vanilla extract

¼ cup dark chocolate chips

¼ cup slivered, toasted almonds

1 Blend almond milk, honey, xanthan gum, almond extract, and vanilla extract together in a blender or by hand.

2 Cover the mixture and refrigerate until completely chilled (about 8 hours or up to 2 days).

3 Freeze the mixture in your ice cream maker according to the manufacturer's instructions.

4 When the sorbet begins to thicken, fold in chocolate chips and almonds and enjoy! If you don't plan on serving the sorbet immediately, transfer to a freezer-proof container and freeze up to 1 week (or 2 months if you use xanthan gum and place a layer of plastic wrap on the surface of the ice cream). To serve, remove from freezer and let sit about 15 minutes, or until desired texture is reached.

How to toast almonds: Spread almonds slivers in an even layer on a baking sheet and then cook at 350°F for 8-10 minutes. If you want your nuts to be evenly toasted, you can redistribute them after 5 minutes.

TROPICAL TWIST SORBET

Tropical Twist Sorbet is also a very good summer flavor. If you want to give your taste buds the island experience, this recipe is for you. Try adding more of your favorite tropical-tasting fruits to diversify this flavor.

YIELD: About 1 quart

1 ⅔ cups reduced-fat coconut milk

4 tablespoons honey

¼ teaspoon xanthan gum (optional)

1 large ginger root, peeled and thinly sliced

1 cup fresh, diced pineapple pieces

1 small banana

¼ medium cucumber

1 In a medium saucepan over low heat, combine the coconut milk, honey, and xanthan gum (if using). Add ginger and let simmer on low until desired strength of flavor is reached, usually about 15 minutes. Once steeped, strain with a fine-mesh strainer to remove ginger slices.

2 Cover the mixture and refrigerate until completely chilled (about 8 hours or up to 2 days).

3 Blend chilled mixture with pineapple, banana, and cucumber in a blender for 30 seconds.

4 Freeze the mixture in your ice cream maker according to the manufacturer's instructions and enjoy! If you don't plan on serving the sorbet immediately, transfer to a freezer-proof container and freeze up to 1 week (or 2 months if you use xanthan gum and place a layer of plastic wrap on the surface of the ice cream). To serve, remove from freezer and let sit about 15 minutes, or until desired texture is reached.

CHAPTER 7: FROZEN CUSTARDS

Custards truly embody the word delectable. The extra egg yolks give them a richer flavor, richer texture, and richer nutrient profile. When you want a dense, full-flavored scoop, go for custard.

TOASTED ALMOND FROZEN CUSTARD

To toast your almond slivers, toss them in a large skillet and cook them on a stovetop over medium heat. Use a heat-resistant spatula or wooden spoon to move them around and keep them from burning. Remove from heat after they start to turn a light shade of brown.

YIELD: About ¾ quart

1 ⅔ cups almond milk

3 tablespoons honey

¼ teaspoon xanthan gum (optional)

½ teaspoon almond extract

2 teaspoons vanilla extract

8 egg yolks

⅓ cup toasted almond slivers

pinch of salt

1   In a medium saucepan over low heat, combine almond milk, honey, xanthan gum (if using), almond extract, and vanilla extract in a medium saucepan over low heat. Stir continuously until the mixture thickens enough to coat the back of a spoon, about 8 minutes. Set aside.

2   In a heat-safe bowl, whisk the egg yolks until they reach a fluffy consistency. Add a small ladle of the warm mixture and stir until combined. Continue adding the warm mixture, one ladle at a time, until it's completely mixed into the egg yolks. Don't add too much of the warm mixture at once or you may end up with scrambled eggs!

3   Cover the mixture and refrigerate until completely chilled (about 8 hours or up to 2 days).

4 Freeze the mixture in your ice cream maker according to the manufacturer's instructions.

5 Midway through the custard's thickening process, sprinkle in toasted almond slivers and salt and enjoy! If you don't plan on serving the custard immediately, transfer to a freezer-proof container and freeze up to 1 week (or 2 months if you use xanthan gum and place a layer of plastic wrap on the surface of the custard). To serve, remove from freezer and let sit about 15 minutes, or until desired texture is reached.

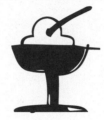

CHOCOLATE MACADAMIA SWIRL FROZEN CUSTARD

Pretty much all nut butters go well with chocolate, so just use your favorite. If swirling in the macadamia nut butter and honey mixture sounds like too much of a challenge, you can drizzle it on your frozen custard after it is already scooped.

YIELD: About ¾ quart

1 ⅔ cups almond milk

3 tablespoons, plus ⅛ cup honey

¼ teaspoon xanthan gum (optional)

1 teaspoon vanilla extract

2 tablespoons cocoa powder

8 egg yolks

¼ cup macadamia nut butter

1 In a medium saucepan over low heat, combine almond milk, 3 tablespoons of honey, xanthan gum (if using), vanilla extract, and cocoa powder. Stir continuously until the mixture thickens enough to coat the back of a spoon, about 8 minutes. Set aside.

2 Whisk egg yolks in a separate bowl. Temper the egg yolks by adding a small ladle of the warm mixture at a time, stirring continuously until completely combined.

3 Cover the mixture and refrigerate until completely chilled (about 8 hours or up to 2 days.)

4 Refrigerate the macadamia nut butter until completely chilled.

5 Freeze the mixture in your ice cream maker according to the manufacturer's instructions.

6 In a medium bowl, combine ⅛ cup honey and macadamia nut butter into one homogeneous mixture and then mix it into the custard

when it is midway through its thickening process and enjoy! If you don't plan on serving the custard immediately, transfer to a freezer-proof container and freeze up to 1 week (or 2 months if you use xanthan gum and place a layer of plastic wrap on the surface of the custard). To serve, remove from freezer and let sit about 15 minutes, or until desired texture is reached.

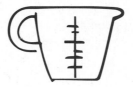

COCONUT CHOCOLATE FROZEN CUSTARD

If you have a real inclination for chocolate and feel cocoa powder isn't enough chocolate for this recipe, worry not. You could also drizzle Chocolate Sauce (page 149) on the ice cream, add homemade Chocolate Pieces (page 148), or do both.

YIELD: About ¾ quart

1 (13.5-ounce) can coconut milk

4 tablespoons honey

¼ teaspoon xanthan gum (optional)

1 cup cream of coconut

8 egg yolks

2 tablespoons cocoa powder

2 tablespoons unsweetened shredded coconut flakes

1 In a medium saucepan over low heat, combine coconut milk, honey, xanthan gum (if using), and cream of coconut. Stir continuously until the mixture thickens enough to coat the back of a spoon, about 8 minutes. Set aside.

2 In a heat-safe bowl, whisk the egg yolks until they reach a fluffy consistency. Add a small ladle of the warm mixture and stir until combined. Continue adding the warm mixture, one ladle at a time, until it's completely mixed into the egg yolks. Don't add too much of the warm mixture at once or you may end up with scrambled eggs!

3 Cover the mixture and refrigerate until completely chilled (about 8 hours or up to 2 days).

4 Blend chilled mixture with cocoa powder and coconut flakes in a blender for 30 seconds.

5 Freeze the mixture in your ice cream maker according to the manufacturer's instructions and enjoy! If you don't plan on serving

the custard immediately, transfer to a freezer-proof container and freeze up to 1 week (or 2 months if you use xanthan gum and place a layer of plastic wrap on the surface of the custard). To serve, remove from freezer and let sit about 15 minutes, or until desired texture is reached.

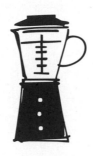

CINNAMON SWIRL FROZEN CUSTARD

Though cinnamon is featured in several other recipes in this book, it deserves its own recipe. Cinnamon used to be valued so highly in ancient times that it was often used as a gift for monarchs. Luckily for us, in this day and age you don't have to be a supreme ruler to get your hands on the delectable spice.

YIELD: About ¾ quart

1 ⅔ cups almond milk

3 tablespoons honey

2 teaspoons vanilla extract

¼ teaspoon xanthan gum (optional)

7 egg yolks

1 tablespoon cinnamon

1 In a medium saucepan over low heat, combine almond milk, honey, vanilla extract, and xanthan gum (if using). Stir continuously until the mixture thickens enough to coat the back of a spoon, about 8 minutes. Set aside.

2 In a heat-safe bowl, whisk the egg yolks until they reach a fluffy consistency. Add a small ladle of the warm mixture and stir until combined. Continue adding the warm mixture, one ladle at a time, until it's completely mixed into the egg yolks. Don't add too much of the warm mixture at once or you may end up with scrambled eggs!

3 Cover the mixture and refrigerate until completely chilled (about 8 hours or up to 2 days).

4 Freeze the mixture in your ice cream maker according to the manufacturer's instructions.

5 As the custard starts to thicken, sprinkle the cinnamon in and enjoy! If you don't plan on serving the ice cream immediately, transfer to a

freezer-proof container and freeze up to 1 week (or 2 months if you use xanthan gum and place a layer of plastic wrap on the surface of the custard). To serve, remove from freezer and let sit about 15 minutes, or until desired texture is reached.

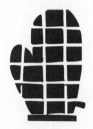

GINGER LEMON FROZEN CUSTARD

This is a very versatile, refreshing dessert. Its flavor is interesting enough to be exciting but isn't so complex that you can only eat it a few times per year.

YIELD: About ¾ quart

1 (13.5-ounce) can coconut milk

4 tablespoons honey

¼ teaspoon xanthan gum (optional)

¼ cup fresh lemon juice

½ cup fresh ginger, peeled and thinly sliced

7 egg yolks

1 In a medium saucepan over low heat, combine coconut milk, honey, xanthan gum (if using), and lemon juice. Add ginger and let simmer on low for 15 minutes or until desired strength of flavor is reached, stirring occasionally. Once steeped, strain with a fine-mesh strainer to remove ginger slices. Set aside.

2 In a heat-safe bowl, whisk the egg yolks until they reach a fluffy consistency. Add a small ladle of the warm mixture and stir until combined. Continue adding the warm mixture, one ladle at a time, until it's completely mixed into the egg yolks.

3 Cover the mixture and refrigerate until completely chilled (about 8 hours or up to 2 days).

4 Freeze the mixture in your ice cream maker according to the manufacturer's instructions. If you don't serve the custard immediately, transfer to a freezer-proof container and freeze up to 1 week (or 2 months if you use xanthan gum and place a layer of plastic wrap on the surface of the custard). To serve, remove from freezer and let sit 15 minutes, or until desired texture is reached.

HOLIDAY SPICE FROZEN CUSTARD

This frozen custard gets its flavor from five spices: star anise, cloves, Chinese cinnamon, Sichuan pepper, and fennel seeds, which makes it a fairly complex flavor, but in no way overpowering.

YIELD: About ¾ quart

1 (13.5-ounce) can coconut milk

3 tablespoons honey

¼ teaspoon xanthan gum (optional)

3 teaspoons Chinese 5-spice powder (ground cinnamon, cloves, star anise, fennel seeds, and Sichuan pepper)

7 egg yolks

1　In a medium saucepan over low heat, combine coconut milk, honey, xanthan gum (if using), and Chinese 5-spice powder. Stir continuously until the mixture thickens enough to coat the back of a spoon, about 8 minutes. Set aside.

2　In a heat-safe bowl, whisk the egg yolks until they reach a fluffy consistency. Add a small ladle of the warm mixture and stir until combined. Continue adding the warm mixture, one ladle at a time, until it's completely mixed into the egg yolks. Don't add too much of the warm mixture at once or you may end up with scrambled eggs!

3　Cover the mixture and refrigerate until completely chilled (about 8 hours or up to 2 days).

4　Freeze the mixture in your ice cream maker according to the manufacturer's instructions. If you don't serve the custard immediately, transfer to a freezer-proof container and freeze up to 1 week (or 2 months if you use xanthan gum and place a layer of plastic wrap on the surface of the custard). To serve, remove from freezer and let sit 15 minutes, or until desired texture is reached.

KAHLÚA ALMOND FUDGE FROZEN CUSTARD

Though White Russian Ice Cream (page 59) is fantastic all by itself, the ante really is upped here with the addition of crunchy almond slivers and chocolaty goodness in the form of Cashew Butter Fudge. If you really want to go crazy with this recipe, you can also add a tablespoon of toasted coconut.

YIELD: About ¾ quart

1 ⅔ cups almond milk

4 tablespoons honey

¼ teaspoon xanthan gum (optional)

8 egg yolks

1 shot of espresso

1 shot of rum

1 teaspoon vanilla extract

½ cup Cashew Butter Fudge (page 152)

¼ cup toasted almond slivers

1 In a medium saucepan over low heat, combine almond milk, honey, and xanthan gum (if using). Stir continuously until the mixture thickens enough to coat the back of a spoon, about 8 minutes. Set aside.

2 In a heat-safe bowl, whisk the egg yolks until they reach a fluffy consistency. Add a small ladle of the warm mixture and stir until combined. Continue adding the warm mixture, one ladle at a time, until it's completely mixed into the egg yolks. Don't add too much of the warm mixture at once or you may end up with scrambled eggs!

3 Cover the mixture and refrigerate until completely chilled (about 8 hours or up to 2 days).

4 Add the espresso, rum, and vanilla extract to the custard mixture and stir until just combined.

5 Freeze the mixture in your ice cream maker according to the manufacturer's instructions.

6 When the custard starts to thicken, make a batch of homemade Cashew Butter Fudge.

7 Pour the not-quite-solidified Cashew Butter Fudge into the ice cream machine along with the toasted almond slivers just before the custard finishes thickening and enjoy! If you don't plan on serving the custard immediately, transfer to a freezer-proof container and freeze up to 1 week (or 2 months if you use xanthan gum and place a layer of plastic wrap on the surface of the custard). To serve, remove from freezer and let sit about 15 minutes, or until desired texture is reached.

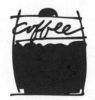

FAUX NUTELLA FROZEN CUSTARD

I'd never been a big Nutella fan before staying with my friend Hauke in Germany, but I left with an appreciation of the spread. If you are a fellow Nutella advocate, you can have the tasty combo of hazelnut and chocolate in your ice cream, too! If you have enjoyed Nutella Fluffernutter sandwiches in the past, you can get something to that effect by subbing cream in for coconut milk.

YIELD: About ¾ quart

1 ⅔ cups almond milk

4 tablespoons honey

¼ teaspoon xanthan gum (optional)

8 egg yolks

¼ cup hazelnut butter

2 tablespoons cocoa powder

1 In a medium saucepan over low heat, combine almond milk, honey, and xanthan gum (if using). Stir continuously until the mixture thickens enough to coat the back of a spoon, about 8 minutes. Set aside.

2 In a heat-safe bowl, whisk the egg yolks until they reach a fluffy consistency. Add a small ladle of the warm mixture and stir until combined. Continue adding the warm mixture, one ladle at a time, until it's completely mixed into the egg yolks. Don't add too much of the warm mixture at once or you may end up with scrambled eggs!

3 Cover the mixture and refrigerate until completely chilled (about 8 hours or up to 2 days).

4 Blend chilled mixture with hazelnut butter and cocoa powder in a blender until a homogeneous texture is achieved, about 30 seconds.

4 Freeze the mixture in your ice cream maker according to the manufacturer's instructions and enjoy! If you don't plan on serving the custard immediately, transfer to a freezer-proof container and freeze up to 1 week (or 2 months if you use xanthan gum and place a layer of plastic wrap on the surface of the custard). To serve, remove from freezer and let sit about 15 minutes, or until desired texture is reached.

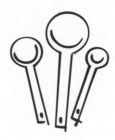

CHAPTER 8: VEGAN ICE CREAMS

Who says you need a milk product to make ice cream!? Using bananas or cashews as a base makes for an interesting alternative to the more traditional ice cream recipes. I omitted the eggs in these recipes because both the banana and cashew provide a thick, creamy texture already which also makes these recipes vegan! Banana- and cashew-based ice cream doesn't exactly taste like something you'd pick up at your local supermarket, but that's part of the fun. The recipes from this chapter should be accepted and enjoyed as their own type of frozen treats. The banana-based recipes are especially great because they don't require the use of an ice cream maker. This saves time and also reduces the amount of dishes that need to be done. There is a small learning curve that involves finding the correctly sized food processor to use, but making banana-based ice cream eventually becomes fast, easy, and, of course, tasty.

CASHEW VANILLA ICE CREAM

Cashews are a naturally creamy nut with a fairly mild taste, so they work surprisingly well as an ice cream base. Here is a good base recipe from which to work.

YIELD: About 1 pint

1 cup cashew butter

3 tablespoons water

⅛ cup honey

2 teaspoons vanilla extract

1 Blend all ingredients in a blender until a smooth, creamy, homogeneous mixture is achieved, about 45 seconds.

2 Transfer mixture to a covered container and refrigerate until completely chilled (about 2 hours or up to 2 days).

3 Freeze mixture in your ice cream maker according to the manufacturer's instructions and enjoy! If you don't plan on serving the ice cream immediately, transfer to a freezer-proof container and freeze up to 1 week. To serve, remove from freezer and let sit about 15 minutes, or until desired texture is reached.

CASHEW STRAWBERRY ICE CREAM

Cashew butter's creamy texture goes well with the sweetness of fresh strawberries. Add a dash of fresh lemon to give it a little more tang.

YIELD: About 1 pint

1 cup cashew butter

3 tablespoons water

⅛ cup honey

1 cup fresh strawberries, hulled

1 Blend all ingredients in a blender until a smooth, creamy, homogeneous mixture is achieved, about 45 seconds.

2 Transfer mixture to a covered container and refrigerate until completely chilled (about 2 hours or up to 2 days).

3 Freeze mixture in your ice cream maker according to the manufacturer's instructions and enjoy! If you don't plan on serving the ice cream immediately, transfer to a freezer-proof container and freeze up to 1 week. To serve, remove from freezer and let sit about 15 minutes, or until desired texture is reached.

BANANA CHIP ICE CREAM

Everybody loves bananas dipped in chocolate. Mix up the classic pairing with banana ice cream and Chocolate Pieces. Put as much or as little chocolate as you like in your ice cream, and you can even add in chocolates of varying sweetness for a more complex flavor.

YIELD: About 1 pint

4 very ripe medium bananas, sliced and frozen

2 teaspoons vanilla extract

½ cup Chocolate Pieces (page 148)

1 Blend bananas and vanilla extract in a food processor or high-powered blender for 3 to 4 minutes or until the mixture becomes smooth and creamy. You might have to push banana pieces down into the mixture if they stick to the sides of your food processor.

2 Fold in Chocolate Pieces and enjoy! If you would like a harder consistency, freeze ice cream in your ice cream maker until desired texture is achieved. If you don't plan on serving the ice cream immediately, transfer to a freezer-proof container and freeze up to 3 days. To serve, remove from freezer and let sit about 10 minutes, or until desired texture is reached.

BANANA ALMOND BUTTER ICE CREAM

If you've only ever eaten peanut butter and almond butter, you should consider trying other nut and seed butters. I personally enjoy macadamia nut butter and hazelnut butter. If you really want to get fancy, you could even try flavored nut/seed butters such as pumpkin spice almond butter or cinnamon vanilla sunflower seed butter. If you like your ice cream pretty sweet, you can add a tablespoon or three of honey in the food processor as well.

YIELD: About 1 pint

4 very ripe medium bananas, sliced and frozen

½ cup almond butter, refrigerated or frozen

pinch of salt

1 Blend all ingredients in a food processor or high-powered blender for 3 to 4 minutes or until the mixture becomes smooth and creamy and enjoy! You might have to push banana pieces down into the mixture if they stick to the sides of your food processor. If you would like a harder consistency, freeze ice cream in your ice cream maker until your desired texture is achieved. If you don't plan on serving the ice cream immediately, transfer to a freezer-proof container and freeze up to 3 days. To serve, remove from freezer and let sit about 10 minutes, or until desired texture is reached.

BANANA NUTELLA ICE CREAM

Bananas taste great. Nutella tastes great. Now imagine these two flavors uniting in ice cream form. It is glorious! Add a tablespoon or 3 of honey in the food processor for extra sweetness.

YIELD: About 1 pint

4 very ripe medium bananas, sliced and frozen

¼ cup hazelnut butter, refrigerated or frozen

2 tablespoons cocoa powder

1 Blend all ingredients in a food processor or high-powered blender for 3 to 4 minutes or until the mixture becomes smooth and creamy and enjoy! You might have to push banana pieces down into the mixture if they stick to the sides of your food processor. If you would like a harder consistency, freeze ice cream in your ice cream maker until your desired texture is achieved. If you don't plan on serving the ice cream immediately, transfer to a freezer-proof container and freeze up to 3 days. To serve, remove from freezer and let sit about 10 minutes, or until desired texture is reached.

PIÑA COLADA ICE CREAM

If you really want to make this taste like the famous drink, add a shot of rum. If you like your ice cream pretty sweet, you can add a tablespoon or 3 of honey in the food processor as well.

YIELD: About 1 pint

4 very ripe medium bananas, sliced and frozen

½ cup frozen coconut milk

½ cup frozen pineapple chunks

1 Blend all ingredients in a food processor or high-powered blender for 3 to 4 minutes or until the mixture becomes smooth and creamy and enjoy! You might have to push banana pieces down into the mixture if they stick to the sides of your food processor. If you would like a harder consistency, freeze ice cream in your ice cream maker until your desired texture is achieved. If you don't plan on serving the ice cream immediately, transfer to a freezer-proof container and freeze up to 3 days. To serve, remove from freezer and let sit about 10 minutes, or until desired texture is reached.

QUICK AND DIRTY BANANA PUMPKIN PIE ICE CREAM

Want the pumpkin pie flavor without the pumpkin pie hassle? Just take some bananas and pumpkin puree out of the freezer and blend 'em! The pumpkin pie spice is a nice touch, and you can add extra cinnamon or nutmeg if you like.

YIELD: About 1 pint

4 very ripe medium bananas, sliced and frozen

¾ cup frozen pumpkin puree

2 teaspoons pumpkin pie spice

1 Blend all ingredients in a food processor or high-powered blender for 3 to 4 minutes or until the mixture becomes smooth and creamy and enjoy! You might have to push banana pieces down into the mixture if they stick to the sides of your food processor. If you would like a harder consistency, freeze ice cream in your ice cream maker until your desired texture is achieved. If you don't plan on serving the ice cream immediately, transfer to a freezer-proof container and freeze up to 3 days. To serve, remove from freezer and let sit about 10 minutes, or until desired texture is reached.

BANANA AVOCADO CHOCOLATE ICE CREAM

Avocado is perhaps the only food that is considered healthy by all nutrition experts. For this reason, many people are always looking for new ways to get avocados into their diet. My favorite way to eat more avocados is by eating. . . ice cream. If you like your ice cream pretty sweet, you can add a tablespoon or 3 of honey in the food processor as well.

YIELD: About 1 pint

4 very ripe medium bananas, sliced and frozen

1 ripe medium avocado, scooped and frozen

1 teaspoon vanilla extract

2 tablespoons cocoa powder

1 Blend all ingredients in a food processor or high-powered blender for 3 to 4 minutes or until the mixture becomes smooth and creamy and enjoy! You might have to push banana pieces down into the mixture if they stick to the sides of your food processor. If you would like a harder consistency, freeze ice cream in your ice cream maker until your desired texture is achieved.

BANANA MINT CHIP ICE CREAM

This is perhaps the most traditional-tasting flavor of the banana recipes because of the peppermint extract. If you like your ice cream pretty sweet, you can add a tablespoon or 3 of honey in the food processor as well.

YIELD: About 1 pint

4 very ripe medium bananas, sliced and frozen

½ ripe medium avocado, scooped and frozen

1 tablespoon peppermint extract

¼ cup Chocolate Pieces (page 148)

1 Blend bananas, avocado, and peppermint extract in a food processor or high-powered blender for 3 to 4 minutes or until the mixture becomes smooth and creamy. You might have to push banana pieces down into the mixture if they stick to the sides of your food processor.

2 Fold in Chocolate Pieces and enjoy! If you would like a harder consistency, freeze ice cream in your ice cream maker until your desired texture is achieved. If you don't plan on serving the ice cream immediately, transfer to a freezer-proof container and freeze up to 3 days. To serve, remove from freezer and let sit about 10 minutes, or until desired texture is reached.

CASHEW CILANTRO LIME ICE CREAM

Cilantro soup is much more common than cilantro ice cream, but on warm days when you want a cool treat instead of hot soup this flavor works splendidly. If you want a normal, familiar ice cream flavor, cashew cilantro lime probably isn't the right choice. But if you want something a bit different and distinct-tasting, this recipe is a good pick!

YIELD: About 1 pint

1 cup cashew butter

1¼ cups plus 1 tablespoon water

⅛ cup honey

pinch of salt

juice of 2 limes

1 very small bunch of cilantro

1 Blend all ingredients in a blender until a smooth, creamy, homogeneous mixture is achieved, about 45 seconds.

2 Transfer mixture to a covered container and refrigerate until completely chilled (about 2 hours or up to 2 days).

3 Freeze mixture in your ice cream maker according to the manufacturer's instructions and enjoy! If you don't plan on serving the ice cream immediately, transfer to a freezer-proof container and freeze up to 1 week. To serve, remove from freezer and let sit about 15 minutes, or until desired texture is reached.

CHAPTER 9: HOMEMADE TOPPINGS AND MORE

People love toppings. A lot. In fact, I think toppings are responsible for the popularity of soft-serve frozen yogurt shops. No one goes out for fro-yo for mediocre-tasting frozen yogurt; they go for the vast assortment of toppings. It is fun to combine different toppings with different flavors of ice cream. More than just fun though, these homemade paleo toppings are absolutely delicious.

CHOCOLATE PIECES

Though there are some good store-bought chocolate options, I prefer making my own chocolate. Coconut oil works well in this recipe, but I also really enjoy making my chocolate with butter. If you want to try using butter, use ½ cup of unsalted butter in place of the coconut oil or use salted butter and nix the extra salt.

YIELD: About 2 cups

½ cup coconut oil

pinch of salt

1 cup cocoa powder

1 teaspoon vanilla extract

⅛ cup honey

1   Melt coconut oil in medium saucepan over low heat.

2   Once coconut oil is completely melted, mix in salt, cocoa powder, vanilla extract, and honey. Stir constantly until a thick, homogeneous texture is achieved, about 30 seconds.

3   Stir the chocolate mixture rapidly for another thirty seconds. Be careful not to overcook, or the chocolate will burn. Remove from heat.

4   While mixture is still warm, spread a very thin layer over a baking sheet lined with wax paper. Let stand in refrigerator or freezer until firm. Once fully chilled, break up the chocolate into small pieces.

SHAVED CHOCOLATE

If you want a more subtle texture to your ice cream, mix in chocolate shavings. Make the chocolate according to the directions above but instead of breaking into pieces, grate the chocolate on a Microplane or cheese grater. For larger shavings, use a vegetable peeler.

CHOCOLATE SAUCE

Chocolate Sauce is a great addition to most ice cream flavors, and this recipe is very simple. Whip it up any time you want to add a little liquid ~~happiness~~ chocolate to your life.

YIELD: About 1 cup

½ cup coconut milk

½ cup cocoa powder

1 teaspoon vanilla extract

1½ tablespoons honey

1 In a medium saucepan stir all ingredients together over low heat until a homogeneous mixture is formed, about 30 seconds.

2 Pour over ice cream and enjoy! If you don't plan on serving sauce immediately, transfer to a covered container and refrigerate up to 2 weeks.

CHOCOLATE SHELL

This is a great recipe to make with kids, because the "magic" shell will harden over the cold ice cream. The coconut oil allows this to happen with its high saturated fat content and tendency to harden at temperatures as high as 77°F. Fun and delicious!

YIELD: About 1 cup

½ cup coconut oil

½ cup cocoa powder

1½ tablespoons honey

1 tablespoon vanilla extract

pinch of sea salt

1   In a medium saucepan stir all ingredients together over low heat until a homogeneous mixture is formed, about 30 seconds.

2   Pour over ice cream and enjoy! If you don't plan on serving sauce immediately, transfer to a covered container and refrigerate up to 2 weeks.

SUNFLOWER SEED BUTTER SAUCE

You can use any number of nut butters in this recipe, and it will still taste great. Adding cocoa powder is also a tasty option if you want a chocolaty flavor.

YIELD: About 1 cup

¼ cup sunflower seed butter

½ cup coconut milk

1½ tablespoons honey

½ teaspoon vanilla extract

pinch of sea salt

1   In a medium saucepan stir all ingredients together over low heat until a homogeneous mixture is formed, about 45 seconds.

2   Pour over ice cream and enjoy! If you don't plan on serving sauce immediately, transfer to a covered container and refrigerate up to 1 week.

CASHEW BUTTER FUDGE

The cashew butter makes for very chewy, yummy fudge. It is fantastic all by itself or as a mix-in to put in your ice cream.

YIELD: About 32 1-inch squares

¼ **cup unsalted butter**

½ **cup cocoa powder**

3 **tablespoons cashew butter**

¼ **teaspoon vanilla extract**

⅛ **teaspoon sea salt**

¼ **cup honey**

1 Melt butter in medium saucepan over low heat.

2 Once butter is completely melted, mix in cocoa powder, cashew butter, vanilla extract, sea salt, and honey. Stir constantly until a thick, homogeneous texture is achieved, about 45 seconds.

3 Stir the fudge mixture rapidly for another thirty seconds. Be careful not to overcook, or the fudge will burn. Remove from heat.

4 While mixture is still warm, spread smoothly over a baking sheet lined with wax paper. Let stand until firm, cut into squares and enjoy! If you don't plan on serving fudge immediately, transfer to a covered container and refrigerate up to 1 week.

FRESH STRAWBERRY SAUCE

This recipe will work wonderfully with other berries, peaches, and mangoes. Of course, if you want to simply place cut-up fruit on your ice cream and skip the pureeing process, that is a great option as well. Berries are my favorite fruit to just plop on ice cream and eat. Delicious, refreshing, and nutritious!

YIELD: About 2 cups

2 cups fresh strawberries, hulled

1 tablespoon honey

½ teaspoon vanilla extract

1   Blend all ingredients in a food processor or high-speed blender.

2   Pour over ice cream and enjoy! If you don't plan on serving sauce immediately, transfer to a covered container and refrigerate for up to 1 week.

BROWNIES

When it comes to this Brownie recipe, no flour means no problem. It is easy to make and fun to eat, and its nutrient content is pretty darn good for a brownie!

YIELD: 9 3-inch squares

1 cup cashew butter

⅓ cup honey

1 egg

2 tablespoons melted butter

1 teaspoon vanilla

⅓ cup cocoa powder

½ teaspoon baking soda

1 Preheat the oven to 325°F.

2 In a large bowl, whisk together the cashew butter, honey, egg, butter, and vanilla until the texture of the mixture is uniform, about 2 minutes.

3 Stir in the cocoa powder and baking soda until homogeneity is again achieved.

4 Pour the batter into an 8 x 8-inch greased baking pan. Bake for 20 to 25 minutes, or until a toothpick comes out clean from the center of the pan.

5 Let cool completely and cut into 3-inch squares.

CARAMEL

I have had the absolute worst luck making caramel. Thank goodness for this recipe! It is so easy a caveman, err, even I can do it. If you are intimidated by making caramel, definitely give this recipe a shot. Not only is it pretty foolproof, but also it tastes amazing.

YIELD: About ½ cup

2 tablespoons water

¼ cup coconut sugar

½ cup coconut milk

1 teaspoon vanilla extract

pinch of salt

1 Place the water and coconut sugar in a small saucepan and bring to a boil over high heat.

2 Add the coconut milk, vanilla extract, and salt and cook for 12 minutes over medium heat. Stir constantly, or the caramel will burn. You'll know your Caramel is done when it becomes thick like jelly and turns dark brown.

COOKIE DOUGH

If you haven't hopped aboard the date cookie train, I would advise you to do so ASAP. Dates give raw, no-bake cookies a fantastic texture and taste. For paleos and nonpaleos alike, this Cookie Dough recipe is to die for!

YIELD: About 12 ½-inch Cookie Dough balls

5 dates

½ cup cashew butter

¼ cup almond flour

½ teaspoon sea salt

1½ teaspoons vanilla extract

¼ cup dark chocolate chips

1 Soak dates for 10 minutes in 2 cups of warm water and then remove pits.

2 Remove dates from the water and then pulse them in a small food processor until smooth.

3 Add cashew butter, almond flour, sea salt, and vanilla extract to food processor and pulse until a homogeneous mixture is formed, about 2 minutes.

4 Fold in chocolate chips.

5 Roll into ½-inch balls and chill in refrigerator. If you don't plan on serving cookie dough immediately, transfer to a covered container and refrigerate for up to 1 week.

CHOCOLATE CHIP COOKIES

Chocolate Chip Cookies are a great complement to ice cream, probably because ice cream has a "milky" component. Break the cookies up and sprinkle them in your ice cream or use them as bookends for your Ice Cream Sandwich (page 165).

YIELD: 8 cookies

3 cups almond flour

1 teaspoon baking soda

1 teaspoon sea salt

⅓ cup honey

1½ teaspoons vanilla extract

2 eggs

½ cup butter

1¼ cups dark chocolate chips

1   Preheat oven to 350°F.

2   In a medium-sized mixing bowl, whisk together almond flour, baking soda, and salt.

3   In a small mixing bowl, whisk together honey, vanilla extract, and eggs.

4   Melt butter and allow it to cool for 5 minutes before whisking it in with the other wet ingredients.

5   Pour wet ingredients into the dry ingredients and then mix them until the dough is completely uniform, about 2 minutes.

4   Add in chocolate chips and then roll the dough into 3-inch balls.

5   Place dough balls on parchment-lined baking sheet with plenty of room between each ball and bake for about 17 minutes and enjoy!

6 If using cookies for an Ice Cream Sandwich, make sure to let them
   cool completely and harden.

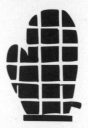

PALEO ICE CREAM

COCONUT SUGAR CONES

Making a homemade cone is not the easiest of tasks, but it is oh-so rewarding. Be patient with this one and bask in the glory of doing something not everyone can say they have done.

YIELD: 8 cones

⅔ cup almond flour

1 tablespoon arrowroot flour

¼ teaspoon salt

4 tablespoons melted palm shortening

2 eggs

½ cup coconut sugar

½ teaspoon vanilla extract

¼ cup coconut milk

1 Preheat the oven to 325°F.

2 In a large mixing bowl, combine the almond flour, arrowroot flour, and salt.

3 Melt the palm shortening in a small saucepan over medium heat.

4 In a small mixing bowl, whisk together the eggs, coconut sugar, vanilla extract, and coconut milk.

5 Let the palm shortening cool for 2 minutes before combining it with the wet mixture.

6 Pour the wet ingredients into the dry ingredients and, using a whisk, mix the two together until the batter is completely smooth.

7 Drop a tablespoon-sized scoop of batter onto the cookie sheet.

8 Smooth the batter into a very thin, approximately 5-inch circle.

9   Bake the large cookie for 15 minutes in the oven, remove from the oven, and roll around an ice cream cone mold. Note that you can make a makeshift mold out of aluminum foil. Make sure to really push down the last edge of the cone so it sticks to the rest of the cone. Also, don't let the cone cool before it is done being rolled.

10 Repeat with the rest of the batter and enjoy! Make as many cones as you can at a time, but making more than a few at once is very difficult because they cool quickly.

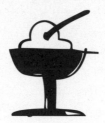

COCONUT WHIPPED CREAM

It is very important that you use full-fat coconut milk for this recipe. The brand you use can cause some variability in the results as well, and from experience I can tell you that Native Forest brand coconut milk works well. If you want to make a primal version of this recipe or if you forgot to pre-chill the coconut milk, you can substitute heavy whipping cream for the coconut, and it will whip very easily.

YIELD: About ½ cup

1 (13.5-ounce) can full-fat coconut milk, chilled overnight

1 teaspoon honey

1 Open the chilled coconut milk and scoop the cream that has risen to the top into a medium-sized bowl. You can save the remaining coconut milk for a smoothie or small batch of ice cream.

2 Using a hand mixer, beat the coconut cream on high for about 3 minutes, drizzling in the honey right as the cream thickens.

3 Top on your favorite ice cream or serve with fresh strawberries. If you don't plan on serving immediately, transfer to a covered container and refrigerate for 3 days.

CHAPTER 10: MORE THAN JUST ICE CREAM

Let's face it, sometimes you want more than a solitary scoop of ice cream. This chapter is full of truly decadent treats for a more novel ice cream experience. Who says eating paleo can't include indulgent treats!? Feel free to mix-and-match with the various recipes throughout this book to give it a more personal touch; the following recipes are merely suggestions.

ICE CREAM SUNDAE

You don't have to use Strawberry Brownie Sundae Ice Cream, Chocolate Sauce, almonds, or even a cherry in this recipe. Use whatever ice cream flavor, type of sauce, nut, and fruit strikes your fancy. Go wild! You could even bake the Chocolate Chip Cookies on the back of a muffin tin to create a chocolate chip cookie bowl.

YIELD: 1 sundae

2 scoops of Strawberry Brownie Sundae Ice Cream (page 84)

¼ cup Chocolate Sauce (page 149)

¼ cup Coconut Whipped Cream (page 161)

⅛ cup toasted, slivered almonds

1 cherry

1 Scoop Strawberry Brownie Sundae Ice Cream into a bowl.

2 Cover your ice cream in Chocolate Sauce.

3 Add a dollop of Coconut Whipped Cream.

4 Sprinkle with toasted almonds.

5 Put a cherry on top of your sundae and enjoy!

ICE CREAM SANDWICH

If you think milk and cookies is a good combination then you really need to try ice cream and cookies. If you don't want to make a sandwich you can simply drop a scoop of ice cream onto a freshly baked cookie. Other ice cream flavors that go particularly well with chocolate chip cookies are Mint Chocolate Chip, Chocolate Chip, Mocha Chip, White Russian, and Cinnamon Swirl.

YIELD: 1 sandwich

2 Chocolate Chip Cookies (page 157)

1 large scoop Vanilla Ice Cream (page 19)

1 Let the ice cream sit out for 15 minutes to soften.

2 Place scoop of ice cream between two cookies. Press down firmly.

KOMBUCHA FLOAT

Soda is clearly off the paleo table, but that doesn't mean ice cream floats have to be. Kombucha makes for a very different float than your standard root beer, but the end result is still a satisfying, fizzy treat.

Other flavors that go well in a kombucha float are Lemon, Watermelon, Blackberry, Mango, and Cherry Vanilla.

Yield: 1 float

1½ cups kombucha

2 scoops Blueberry Ice Cream (page 46)

1 Pour the kombucha in a large glass or mug, drop the ice cream in, and enjoy immediately.

AFFOGATO

Affogato means "drowned" in Italian, and it is a must-try for coffee lovers. You can eat the ice cream and then drink the leftover coffee at the end or mix the ice cream into the coffee and then enjoy a sweet, creamy coffee drink. *Evviva!*

YIELD: 1 dessert

2 scoops Vanilla Ice Cream (page 19)

1½ cups of very strongly brewed coffee

1 Place ice cream in a large glass or mug, pour hot coffee over ice cream, and enjoy immediately.

ICE POPS

On the truly hot days, ice cream might not be enough to fend off the heat. For these scorching days, make some sorbet Popsicles and cool off. If you want your Popsicles to be a bit creamier, you can use regular ice cream recipes to make them. If you are a really big Popsicle fan, you can even buy dedicated ice pop molds.

YIELD: about ¾ quart or 14 ice pops

1 batch of any sorbet flavor*

*Note: Make sure you don't put your mixture into an ice cream maker before making ice pops.

1 Follow the instructions provided for making the sorbet of your choice. Do not put the mixture in the ice cream maker—leave in liquid form.

2 Pour the sorbet mixture into an ice pop tray, small, plastic cups, or an ice cube tray that makes very large cubes.

3 Place aluminum foil or plastic wrap over the top of the cups.

4 Poke Popsicle sticks through the aluminum foil to the bottom of the cups. The aluminum foil will hold the sticks in place.

5 Put your Popsicles in the freezer.

6 Once your Popsicles are good and frozen, remove the aluminum foil and place the cups in a shallow bowl of water for a few minutes.

7 Carefully remove your Popsicles and enjoy!

FUDGE BARS

If you want your fudge bar to be extra rich, add a few extra egg yolks. For a refreshing twist to the classic fudge bar, try adding ½ tablespoon of raspberry puree to each bar right as it begins to harden. Fudge bars were one of my go-to picks from the ice cream truck, and I have to say making them at home is more convenient than chasing after the ice cream man in bare feet on hot pavement.

YIELD: About ¾ quart or 14 fudge bars

1 batch Chocolate Ice Cream (page 16)*

> *Note: Make sure you don't put your mixture into an ice cream maker before making ice pops.

1 Follow instructions 1–3 of the Chocolate Ice Cream recipe.

1 Pour the ice cream mixture into an ice pop tray, small, plastic cups, or an ice cube tray that makes very large cubes.

2 Place aluminum foil or plastic wrap over the top of the cups.

3 Poke Popsicle sticks through the aluminum foil to the bottom of the cups. The aluminum foil will hold the sticks in place.

4 Put your fudge bars in the freezer.

5 Once your fudge bars are good and frozen, remove the aluminum foil and place the cups into a shallow bowl of water for a few minutes.

6 Carefully remove your fudge bars and enjoy!

LAST THOUGHTS

If you give a man a fish, you'll feed him for a day. If you teach a man to fish, you'll feed him for a lifetime. Or until the lake freezes over, at least; then you'll need to teach him to hunt.

I hope I've given you enough of a start so that you can now enjoy homemade, nutritious ice cream for the rest of your life. The intent of this book was not to give you 75 flavors from which to choose. Rather, it was to show you my favorite recipes and give you the ability to tweak them or even come up with something radically different. Each of us is unique and has our own set of taste buds and preferences.

Make ice cream that you love. Use nourishing ingredients. Share with family and friends. And remember to enjoy every bite!

CONVERSIONS

USEFUL CONVERSIONS

U.S. MEASURE	EQUIVALENT	METRIC
1 teaspoon	—	5 milliliters
1 tablespoon	3 teaspoons	15 milliliters
1 cup	16 tablespoons	240 milliliters
1 pint	2 cups	470 milliliters
1 quart	4 cups	950 milliliters
1 liter	4 cups + 3½ tablespoons	1000 milliliters
1 ounce (dry)	2 tablespoons	28 grams
1 pound	16 ounces	450 grams
2.21 pounds	35.3 ounces	1 kilogram
270°F / 350°F	—	132°C / 177°C

VOLUME CONVERSIONS

U.S. MEASURE	EQUIVALENT	METRIC
1 tablespoon	½ fluid ounce	15 milliliters
¼ cup	2 fluid ounces	60 milliliters
⅓ cup	3 fluid ounces	90 milliliters
½ cup	4 fluid ounces	120 milliliters
⅔ cup	5 fluid ounces	150 milliliters
¾ cup	6 fluid ounces	180 milliliters
1 cup	8 fluid ounces	240 milliliters
2 cups	16 fluid ounces	480 milliliters

WEIGHT CONVERSIONS

U.S. MEASURE	METRIC
1 ounce	30 grams
⅓ pound	150 grams
½ pound	225 grams
1 pound	450 grams

RECIPE INDEX

ACKNOWLEDGMENTS

Thanks to Barefoot Ted, whose Google group led me to the paleo framework and ultimately jump-started my interest in nutrition.

Thanks to my parents, Rich and Wendi, and my girlfriend, Kelsey, for really being there for me.

Thanks to Loren Cordain, Chris Kresser, Mark Sisson, Robb Wolf, and everyone else who has spearheaded the ancestral health movement.

Thanks to Kelly Reed for reaching out to me about the possibility of acquiring this book.

ABOUT THE AUTHOR

BEN HIRSHBERG is a student, author, and entrepreneur who studies the art of living well. Born and bred in Seattle, Washington, Ben likes to read, cook, run, travel, and throw convivial parties. Ben has Personal Fitness Trainer, Youth Exercise Specialist, and Fitness Nutrition Specialist certifications through the World Instructor Training School and the National Academy of Sports Medicine and is in the process of becoming a nutritional therapy practitioner and achieving board certification in Holistic Nutrition by the National Association of Nutrition Professionals. He also writes regular articles for *Paleo Magazine* and irregular articles for various websites. Ben runs his personal website at www.BenHirshberg.com and offers a free eBook to his mailing list subscribers.